without the | takeaway
the | favourites
calories | Justine Pattison

Low-calorie recipes, cheats and ideas
from around the world

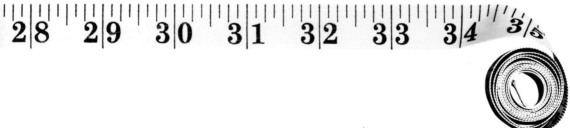

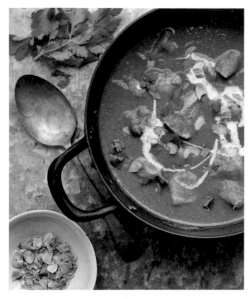

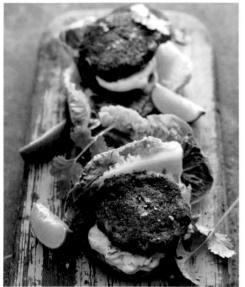

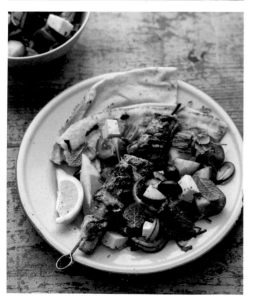

contents

introduction 5

without the calories | takeaway favourites

the

Justine Pattison

For John, Jess and Emily

introduction

MY STORY

I struggled with my weight for years. After being a skinny child and teenager, I piled on the weight during my last years of school and went into my twenties feeling fat and frumpy. A career as a cookery writer and food stylist has helped me understand good food but because my kitchen is always overflowing with great things to eat, temptation is never far away. My weight yo-yoed for twenty years and at my heaviest I weighed more than 15 stone.

A few years ago, I worked on the hit TV series *You Are What You Eat* – I put together those groaning tables of bad food. I also had the chance to work with the contributors on the show, guiding them through the dieting process and helping them discover a whole new way of eating and cooking. Having been overweight myself, I became passionate about helping people lose weight.

Since then, I've worked as a food consultant on many of the weight loss shows you've seen on TV, and written diet plans and recipes for best-selling books, newspapers and magazines. I'm so proud that thousands of people have successfully followed my way of cooking and lost weight.

This book, and the others in the *Without the Calories* series, are ideal for anyone who wants to lose weight while leading a normal life. Cooking these recipes will help you sustain a happy, healthy weight loss. That's what it's all about: you don't have to be stick thin, but you deserve to feel good about yourself. My *Without the Calories* recipes will help you reach your goal.

ABOUT THIS BOOK

It's rare to find someone who doesn't love a rich, spicy curry, a crisp pizza oozing with melted cheese or piping hot fish and chips straight out of the fryer, and our high streets are teeming with takeaway restaurants offering dishes for instant gratification. But if you're already carrying more weight than you'd like, or simply want to eat more healthily, takeaway food can be a nutritional disaster.

In this book, I've picked popular takeaway dishes and reworked the ingredients and cooking methods to cut the calories and help you lose weight in the most delicious and simple way possible. You'll find everything from a creamy chicken korma to super-quick pizzas and succulent burgers, all given a low-calorie workout without losing their appeal.

I'm not going to make rash promises about how many pounds my alternative recipes will help you shed, but I do know that when it comes to losing weight, finding foods that give you pleasure and fit into your lifestyle are the key to success. When you eat well without obsessing over rapid weight loss, it's easier to relax and lose what you need to comfortably – and safely.

To help everyone enjoy these reinvented dishes, I've used easy-to-find ingredients and given clear, simple cooking instructions. There's lots of freezer information included, so you know which dishes you can store safely for another day.

If you're already following a diet plan, you'll find additional nutritional information at the back of the book that'll help you work my recipes into your week. And, if you're stuck for inspiration and have a few pounds to lose, try my 123 Plan – it couldn't be easier.

USING THE 123 PLAN

If you're not following a diet regime at the moment and want a great kick-start, try my 123 Plan for a few weeks. I've tried to make it really easy, and you don't need to do too much adding up. Just pick one recipe from any section to bring your daily intake to between 900 and 1,200 calories. Add an *essential extra* 300 calories a day and you'll be on your way to a healthy, sustainable weight loss of between 2–3lbs a week.

ONE
up to 300 calories

TWO
300–400 calories

THREE
400–500 calories

YOUR ESSENTIAL EXTRAS

These extra 300 calories can be made up of accompaniments, such as potatoes, rice and pasta, as well as snacks or treats; there are suggestions and serving sizes on page 180. You'll also find recipes that contain under 200 calories per portion, which can be included as part of your essential extras. As long as your extras don't exceed 300 calories a day, you'll be on track.

WHEN TO EAT

The 123 Plan is flexible, so if you find you fancy a **ONE** or **TWO** recipe rather than a **THREE** as your third meal of the day, just add enough calories to bring it into the right range. Don't worry if the calculations aren't absolutely accurate – a difference of 25 or less calories per serving won't affect your weekly allowance.

You don't have to eat your lightest meal for breakfast and the most calorific meal late in the day – in fact, the opposite often works best. I tend to eat my largest meal at lunchtime if I can, and have a lighter meal in the evening, but work with what suits you and your family best.

If you want to add your own favourite meals into the plan, just make sure they are within the recommended calorie boundaries and calculate accordingly. (You may find this useful when planning breakfast especially.)

DON'T RUSH IT

Weight tends to be gained over time, and losing it gradually will make the process easier and help give your body, especially your skin, time to adapt. You're more likely to get into positive, enjoyable long-term cooking and eating habits this way too.

WHAT IS A CALORIE?

Put simply, a calorie is a unit of energy contained within food and drink which our bodies burn as fuel. Different foods contain varying amounts of calories and if more calories are consumed than the body needs, the excess will be stored as fat. To lose weight, we need to eat less or use more energy by increasing our activity – and ideally both!

I've provided the calorie content of a single serving of each dish. In my experience, most people will lose at least 2lb a week by consuming around 1,200–1,500 calories a day, but it's always best to check with your GP before you start a new regime. Everyone is different and, especially if you have several stones to lose, you'll need some personalised advice. The calories contained in each recipe have been calculated as accurately as possible, but could vary a little depending on your ingredients.

A few wayward calories here and there won't make any difference to your overall weight loss.

If you have a couple of days of eating more than 1,400 calories, try to eat closer to 1,100 for the next few days. Over a week, things will even out.

My recipes strike a balance between eating and cooking well and reducing calories, and I've tried them all as part of my own way of enjoying food without putting on excess weight. Even if you don't need to lose weight, I hope you enjoy cooking from my books simply because you like the recipes.

SECRETS OF SUCCESS

The serving sizes that I've recommended form the basis of the nutritional information on page 182, and if you eat any more, you may find losing weight takes longer. If you're cooking for anyone who doesn't need to watch their calorie intake, simply increase their servings and offer plenty of accompaniments.

The right portion size also holds the key to maintaining your weight loss. Use this opportunity to get used to smaller servings. Work out exactly how much food your body needs to maintain the shape that makes you feel great. That way, even when counting calories feels like a distant memory, you'll remain in control of your eating habits.

Stick to lean protein (which will help you feel fuller for longer) and vegetables and avoid high-fat, high-sugar snacks and confectionery. Be aware that alcohol is packed with empty calories and could weaken your resolve. Starchy carbs such as pasta, rice, potatoes and bread are kept to a minimum because I've found that, combined with eating lots of veg and good protein, this leads to more sustainable weight loss. There's no need to avoid dairy products such as cheese and cream, although they tend to be high in fat and calories. You can swap the high-fat versions for reduced-fat ones, or use less.

Ditch heavily processed foods and you will feel so much better. Switching to more natural ingredients will help your body work with you.

Most recipes here form the main part of each meal, so there's room to have your plate half-filled with freshly cooked vegetables or a colourful, crunchy salad. This will help fill you up, and boost your intake of vitamins and minerals.

Make sure you drink enough fluids, especially water – around 2 litres is ideal. Staying hydrated will help you lose weight more comfortably, and it's important when you exercise too.

IN THE KITCHEN

Pick up some electronic kitchen scales and a set of measuring spoons if you don't already have them. Both will probably cost less than a takeaway meal for two, and will help ensure good results.

Invest, if you can, in a large, deep non-stick frying pan and a medium non-stick saucepan. The non-stick coating means that you will need less oil to cook, and a frying pan with a wide base and deep sides can double as a wok.

I use oil and butter sparingly, and use a calorie-controlled spray oil for frying. I also keep a jam jar with a little sunflower oil and a heatproof pastry brush for greasing pans lightly before frying. See page 176 for more information on ingredients and equipment.

STICK WITH IT

Shifting your eating habits and trying to lose weight is not easy, especially if you have been eating the same way for many years. But it isn't too late. You may never have the perfect body, but you can have one that, fuelled by really good food, makes you feel happy and healthy. For more information and menu plans visit www. justinepattison.co.uk.

Enjoy!

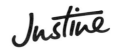

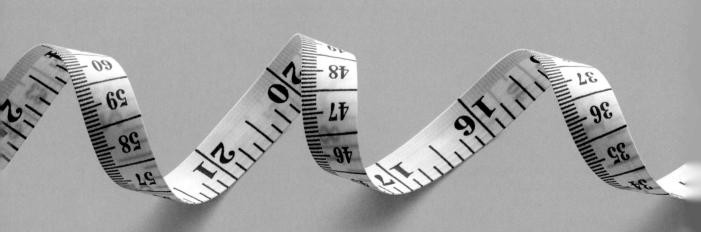

indian

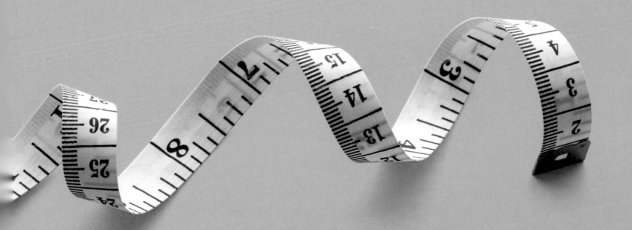

210
CALORIES
PER SERVING

tandoori chicken

SERVES 4
PREP: 5–10 MINUTES,
PLUS MARINATING TIME
COOK: 8 MINUTES

4 boneless, skinless chicken
    breasts (each about 175g)
minted yoghurt sauce (see
    page 40), to serve
lemon wedges, for
    squeezing

FOR THE MARINADE
1 tbsp garam masala
1 tbsp Kashmiri chilli powder
25g chunk fresh root ginger,
    peeled and finely grated
4 garlic cloves, crushed
150g fat-free natural
    yoghurt
1 tbsp fresh lemon juice
¼ tsp cayenne pepper
1 tsp fine sea salt

Freeze the cooked and
cooled chicken pieces in
a zip-seal bag for up to
1 month. Thaw in the
fridge overnight. Reheat
in the microwave or a
moderate oven until
piping hot.

These chicken breast pieces are not only packed with flavour
on their own, but the yoghurt marinade makes them tender
and juicy too. Kashmiri chilli powder gives the chicken a lovely
red colour, but you can also use a mixture of 2 teaspoons of
paprika and 1 teaspoon of hot chilli powder, which will work
just as well. Serve with a large, colourful salad.

To make the marinade, put all the ingredients in a large
non-metallic bowl and mix together well.

Put the chicken on a board, cut the pieces in half and then
slash each piece 3–4 times with a knife. Put the chicken in
the marinade and turn over to coat it. Cover with cling film
and leave to marinate in the fridge for 1–4 hours or overnight.

Preheat the grill to its hottest setting. Line a baking tray or
grill pan with foil and place a rack on top. Take the chicken
pieces from the marinade, shaking off any excess, and place
them on the rack.

Cook the chicken under the hot grill, fairly close to the element
so the chicken chars, for about 8 minutes on each side. Check
the chicken is cooked by piercing it with the tip of a knife and
having a look inside – there should be no pink remaining. (You
can also bake the chicken at 200°C/Fan 180°C/Gas 6 for 16–20
minutes, but you won't get the authentic-looking charred bits.)

Serve the tandoori chicken hot or cold with minted yoghurt
sauce (see page 40) and lemon wedges for squeezing over.

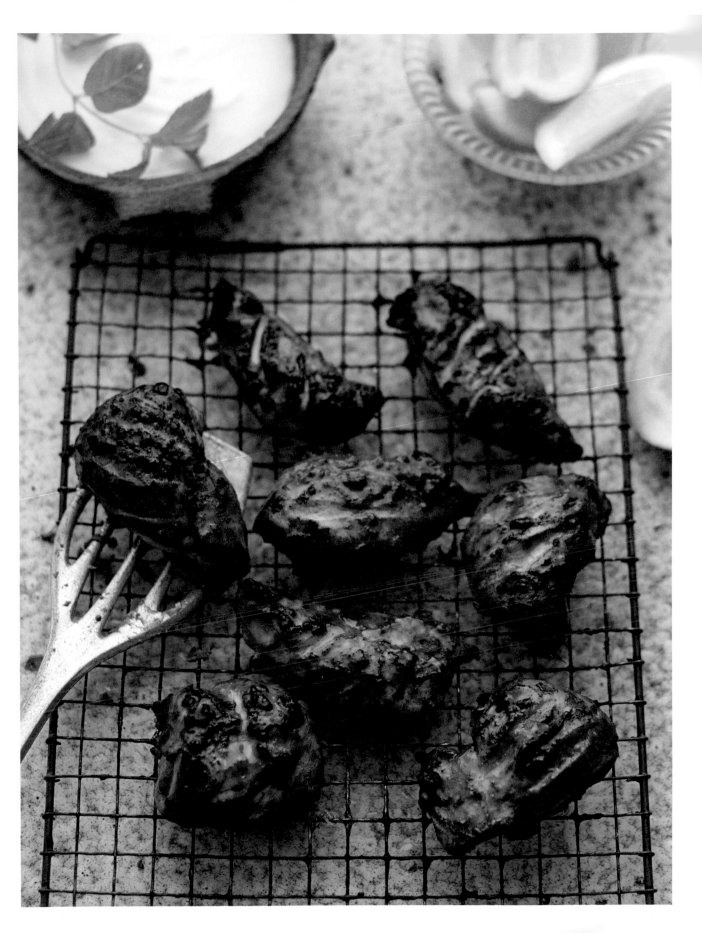

291
CALORIES
PER SERVING

my favourite chicken tikka masala

SERVES 4

PREP: 15 MINUTES, PLUS MARINATING TIME

COOK: 40 MINUTES

4 boneless, skinless chicken breasts
1 tsp sunflower oil

FOR THE MARINADE
2 tbsp medium curry powder
2 tsp smoked paprika (not hot smoked)
1 tsp flaked sea salt
100g fat-free natural yoghurt

FOR THE SAUCE
1 tbsp sunflower oil
2 large onions, chopped
4 garlic cloves, sliced
25g chunk fresh root ginger, peeled and finely grated
4 tsp medium curry powder
2 tbsp tomato purée
1 tsp caster sugar
1 tsp flaked sea salt
400ml cold water
15g fresh coriander, leaves finely chopped
2 tbsp double or single cream (optional)

Freeze the cooled curry in a zip-seal bag or in foil containers for up to 3 months. Thaw in the fridge overnight. Reheat thoroughly in a large, wide-based saucepan, stirring gently until piping hot.

This recipe has a rich sauce but is actually pretty low in fat and calories. Cooking the marinated chicken in a dry pan before adding the sauce gives it a lovely charred flavour, very close to what you might expect from a proper tandoor oven. Stir in a little cream if you like your curries richer, but remember to add the extra calories to each serving.

Cut the chicken into roughly 3cm chunks. To make the marinade, mix the curry powder, paprika and salt in a large bowl. Add the yoghurt and stir until well combined. Stir the chicken pieces into the marinade and mix until well coated. Cover and leave to marinate in the fridge for 1–4 hours. The yoghurt will help tenderise the chicken pieces.

While the chicken is marinating, make the sauce. Heat the oil in a large non-stick saucepan and add the onions, garlic and ginger. Cover and cook over a low heat for 15 minutes or until very soft and lightly coloured. Remove the lid and stir the onions occasionally so they don't begin to stick.

Add the curry powder to the pan and cook uncovered for 1 minute, stirring. Add the tomato purée, caster sugar and salt and fry for a few seconds more, stirring constantly.

Pour the water into the pan and simmer the sauce gently for 10 minutes, stirring occasionally. Remove the pan from the heat and use a stick blender to blitz the sauce until it is as smooth as possible. Set aside.

Heat the teaspoon of oil into a large non-stick frying pan and fry the marinated chicken pieces for about 6 minutes over a medium-high heat, turning occasionally until lightly charred on most sides – this will help give the curry an authentic flavour.

Gently add the chicken pieces to the masala sauce – watch out for splashes – and stir in the coriander and cream, if using. Simmer gently for 4 minutes more or until the chicken is tender and cooked through, stirring regularly.

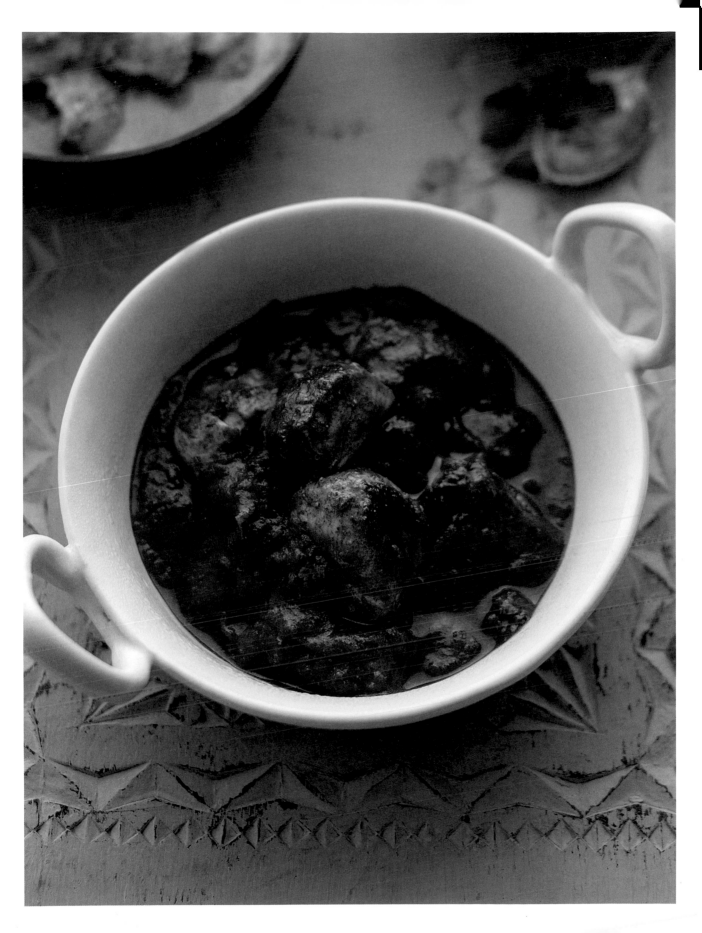

297

creamy chicken passanda

SERVES 6
PREP: 20 MINUTES,
PLUS MARINATING TIME
COOK: 50–55 MINUTES

1kg boneless, skinless
   chicken thighs (around 10)
1 tbsp sunflower oil
2 large onions, thinly sliced
8 cardamom pods, lightly
   crushed
2 tsp fenugreek seeds
1 tbsp garam masala
2 tbsp ground almonds
2 tsp caster sugar
1½ tsp flaked sea salt, plus
   extra to season
¼ tsp ground cinnamon
350ml cold water
2 tsp dried fenugreek leaves
3 tbsp double cream
ground black pepper
fresh coriander leaves,
   to garnish (optional)

FOR THE MARINADE
200g fat-free natural
   yoghurt
20g chunk of fresh root
   ginger, peeled and
   roughly chopped
4 garlic cloves, peeled
2 tsp ground cumin
1 tsp ground coriander
1 tsp ground turmeric
¼ tsp hot chilli powder

Freeze the cooled curry
in a zip-seal bag or in foil
containers for up to 3 months.
Thaw in the fridge overnight.
Reheat thoroughly in a large,
wide-based saucepan, stirring
gently until piping hot.

This lightly spiced sauce contains methi, or fenugreek leaves, which make all the difference in adding authenticity. You'll find them in larger supermarkets and Asian food stores. You can add 3 tablespoons of chopped fresh coriander leaves if you can't find methi and the curry will still be delicious.

Put all the ingredients for the marinade in a food processor or blender and blitz until the mixture is smooth. Scrape into a large non-metallic bowl. Trim the chicken thighs, removing any visible fat with kitchen scissors. Cut each thigh into 3 pieces and stir into the marinade. Cover and leave in the fridge for 1–4 hours.

To make the sauce, heat the oil in a large flameproof casserole or non-stick saucepan over a low heat. Stir in the onions, cover, and fry gently for 10 minutes or until well softened. Remove the lid every now and then and stir so the onions don't begin to stick. After 10 minutes, remove the lid, turn up the heat a little and fry for a further 5 minutes until lightly browned, stirring.

Take the pan off the heat and blitz the onions with a stick blender until they are as smooth as possible. (Alternatively, let the onions cool for a few minutes and transfer them to a food processor for blending, then return them to the pan.)

Return the pan to the heat and add the cardamom pods, fenugreek seeds and garam masala to the onions. Cook for 2 minutes, stirring continuously then add the chicken and marinade to the pan. Cook over a medium heat for 2–3 minutes, stirring continuously. Add the ground almonds, sugar, salt, cinnamon and cold water. Sprinkle the fenugreek leaves on top, stir well and bring to a gentle simmer.

Cover the pan loosely with a lid and leave to simmer for 25–30 minutes or until the chicken is very tender and the sauce is beginning to thicken, stirring occasionally.

Stir in the double cream and increase the heat. Simmer for 8–10 minutes or until the sauce is thick, stirring regularly. Season with salt and pepper and serve garnished with coriander, if using.

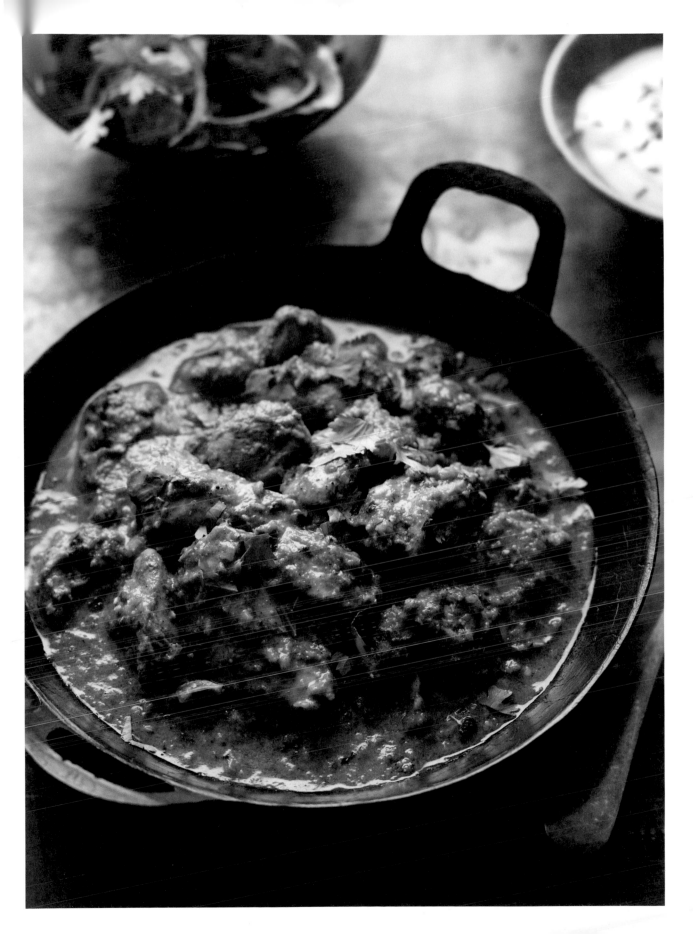

279
CALORIES
PER SERVING

chicken jalfrezi

SERVES 4
PREP: 20 MINUTES
COOK: 20 MINUTES

4 long green chillies
4 boneless, skinless
  chicken breasts
4 tsp sunflower oil
500g ripe tomatoes,
  roughly chopped
3 garlic cloves, finely
  chopped
2 tsp ground cumin
2 tsp garam masala
1 tsp hot chilli powder
1 tbsp caster sugar
1 tsp flaked sea salt
1 medium onion,
  cut into 12 wedges
1 green and 1 red pepper,
  deseeded and cut
  into 3cm chunks
175ml cold water

Freeze the cooled curry
in a zip-seal bag or in
foil containers for up to
3 months. Thaw in the
fridge overnight. Reheat
thoroughly in a large, wide-
based saucepan, stirring
gently until piping hot.

This is a colourful, medium-hot curry with a rich tomato sauce. For a milder curry, leave out the chilli powder and rely on the heat from the chillies. If you can't find the long green chillies, use the plump ones or opt for the riper red ones instead.

Place the chillies on a board and finely chop 2 of them. (Deseed the chillies first if you don't like your curries too hot and spicy.) Split the other 2 from stalk to tip on one side without opening them or removing the seeds. Cut each chicken breast into roughly 3cm chunks.

Heat 2 teaspoons of the oil in a large wok or deep, non-stick frying pan over a high heat. Add the chopped tomatoes, garlic, chopped chillies, cumin, garam masala, chilli powder, sugar and salt. Cook for 5 minutes, stirring regularly, or until the tomatoes soften into a thick sauce.

While the sauce is simmering, heat the remaining oil in a large frying pan and stir-fry the chicken, onion and peppers for 3–4 minutes or until lightly browned.

Add the browned chicken pieces, onions and peppers and the whole chillies to the spicy tomato sauce. Pour over the cold water and reduce the heat slightly. Return to a simmer and cook for 8–10 minutes or until the chicken is tender and cooked through, stirring occasionally.

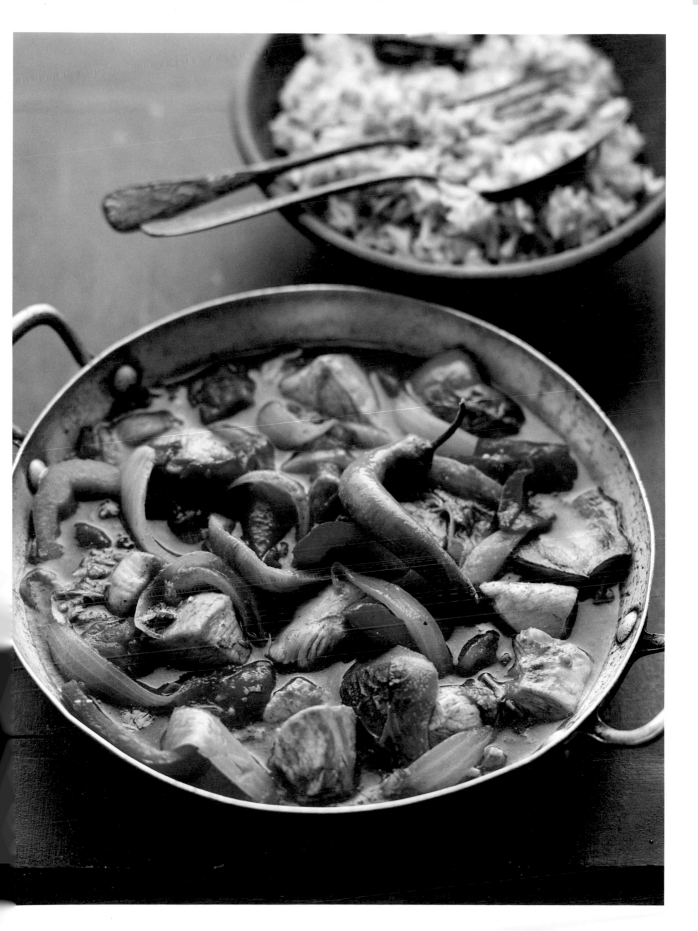

323
CALORIES
PER SERVING

chicken korma

SERVES 4
PREP: 15 MINUTES,
PLUS MARINATING TIME
COOK: 45 MINUTES

4 boneless, skinless
   chicken breasts
3 tbsp fat-free natural
   yoghurt
oil, for spraying or brushing
ground black pepper

FOR THE SAUCE
1 tbsp sunflower oil
2 large onions, chopped
4 garlic cloves, sliced
25g chunk of fresh root
   ginger, peeled and
   finely grated
3 tbsp korma curry paste
   (or any mild curry paste)
2 tsp caster sugar
1 tsp flaked sea salt,
   plus extra to season
400ml cold water

TO SERVE
3 tbsp single cream
fresh coriander leaves,
   to garnish (optional)
1–2 tsp toasted almond
   flakes (optional)

Freeze the cooled curry
in a zip-seal bag or in
foil containers for up to
3 months. Thaw in the
fridge overnight. Reheat
thoroughly in a large, wide-
based saucepan, stirring
gently until piping hot.

Make sure you use a korma paste and not a ready-made korma sauce for this dish as the results will be very different. Curry pastes sometimes have a layer of oil on the surface, so I drain that off to reduce the calorie count even further.

Cut each chicken breast into roughly 3cm chunks and put in a large bowl. Season with black pepper and stir in the yoghurt. Cover and leave to marinate in the fridge for 1–4 hours. The yoghurt will help tenderise the chicken pieces.

To make the sauce, heat the oil in a large, non-stick saucepan and add the onions, garlic and ginger. Cover and cook over a low heat for 15 minutes or until very soft and lightly coloured. Remove the lid every now and then and give the onions a stir so they don't begin to stick to the bottom of the pan.

Once the onions are softened, stir in the curry paste, sugar and salt. Cook for 1 minute, stirring constantly. Slowly pour the cold water into the pan, stirring constantly. Bring to a gentle simmer, then cover and cook for 15 minutes, stirring occasionally.

Remove the pan from the heat and blitz the onion mixture with a stick blender until it is as smooth as possible. (If you don't have a stick blender, leave the mixture to cool for a few minutes then transfer it to a food processor and blitz to a purée.) This sauce can now be set aside until the chicken has finished marinating, so allow it to cool, then cover and chill.

Spray or brush a large non-stick frying pan with oil and place over a medium heat. Fry the chicken for 5 minutes or until lightly coloured on all sides, turning regularly. Pour the cooked sauce over the chicken and bring to a gentle simmer.

Cook the chicken for 6–8 minutes or until tender and cooked through, stirring regularly. Adjust the seasoning to taste and drizzle with the cream. Scatter fresh coriander on top and toasted almond flakes, if using.

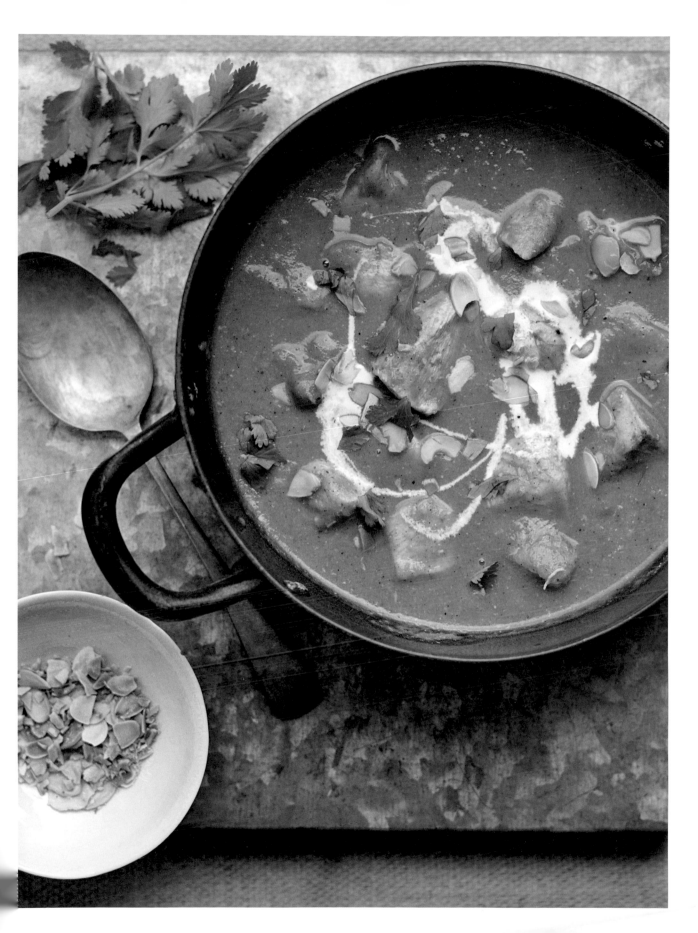

375

CALORIES
PER SERVING

lamb rogan josh

SERVES 6
PREP: 20 MINUTES
COOK: 2–2¼ HOURS

1 tbsp sunflower oil
2 medium onions,
  thinly sliced
1.2kg lean lamb leg steaks
  (or boneless lamb leg)
3 plump red chillies, finely
  chopped (deseeded if
  you like)
4 garlic cloves, finely
  chopped
25g chunk fresh root ginger,
  peeled and finely grated
2 tsp paprika (not smoked)
2 tsp garam masala
1 tsp ground coriander
1 tsp fennel seeds
1 tsp cumin seeds
½ tsp hot chilli powder
2 x 400g cans chopped
  tomatoes
200ml cold water
2 bay leaves
1 cinnamon stick
20g fresh coriander,
  roughly chopped,
  including the stalks
200g young spinach leaves
flaked sea salt
ground black pepper

Freeze the cooled curry
in a zip-seal bag or in
foil containers for up to
3 months. Thaw in the
fridge overnight. Reheat
thoroughly in a large, wide-
based saucepan, stirring
gently until piping hot.

This might look like a huge number of ingredients for one curry, but the end result is well worth the effort. The spices are all readily available in most supermarkets and will last for months in the cupboard so they won't go to waste.

Heat the oil in a large flameproof casserole. Add the onions and cook over a low heat for 15 minutes or until well softened and golden brown, stirring regularly. Richly coloured onions will add lots of flavour to the curry but they mustn't burn, so keep a good eye on them. If the onions start to stick, simply add a splash of water and continue cooking.

Preheat the oven to 180°C/Fan 160°C/Gas 4. Trim the lamb steaks of any hard fat and cut into roughly 3cm chunks. Season with salt and lots of black pepper.

Add the chopped chillies, garlic and ginger to the onions and cook together for 2 minutes, stirring with a wooden spoon. Stir in the lamb and cook for 3–4 minutes, turning regularly, or until lightly coloured on all sides.

Sprinkle over the paprika, garam masala, ground coriander, fennel and cumin seeds and chilli powder and stir well. Cook for a further 2 minutes, stirring and adding a little water if the spices begin to stick to the bottom of the pan.

Tip the canned tomatoes into the dish and add the water, bay leaves, cinnamon stick and chopped coriander. Stir well, bring to a simmer and cover with a lid. Transfer to the oven and cook for about 1½ hours or until the lamb is very tender and the sauce is thick. Check the curry after an hour if you can, and give it a gentle stir. It's important not to stir too much as the lamb pieces could break up.

Take the curry out of the oven and remove the lid. Stir in the spinach, a handful at a time, then return the dish to the oven for 10 minutes, which should be long enough for the spinach to soften and wilt into the curry. Add a little more salt and pepper to taste just before serving.

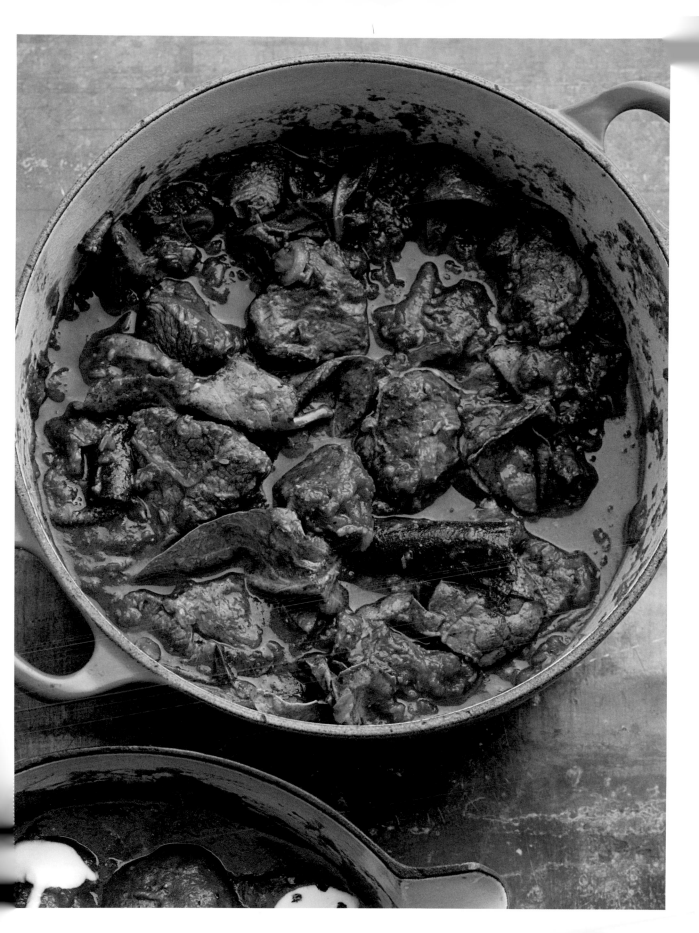

335
CALORIES
PER SERVING

lamb meatball curry

SERVES 4
**PREP: 20 MINUTES,
PLUS CHILLING TIME**
COOK: 50-60 MINUTES

450g lean minced lamb
1 medium onion, finely
  chopped
2 garlic cloves, crushed
finely grated zest of 1 lemon
2 tsp garam masala
15g fresh mint leaves,
  finely chopped
1 tsp flaked sea salt,
  plus extra to season
ground black pepper
oil, for spraying or brushing
2 tbsp fat-free natural
  yoghurt, to serve

FOR THE SAUCE
2 tsp sunflower oil
2 medium onions,
  thinly sliced
4 garlic cloves, thinly sliced
20g chunk fresh root ginger,
  peeled and finely chopped
¼–½ tsp hot chilli powder
1 tbsp garam masala
680ml jar or carton passata
  (sieved Italian tomatoes)
500ml lamb stock (made
  with ½ lamb stock cube)

Freeze the cooled curry
in a zip-seal bag or in
foil containers for up to
3 months. Thaw in the
fridge overnight. Reheat
thoroughly in a large, wide-
based saucepan, stirring
gently until piping hot.

These spicy meatballs taste wonderfully comforting and authentic. If you can't find passata, use 2 x 400g of canned chopped tomatoes instead. You can also have the meatballs without the sauce, served warm or cold with a salad, or packed into pitta bread (but they will need frying for a few minutes longer so they are cooked through).

To make the meatballs, mix the lamb mince in a large bowl with the onion, garlic, lemon zest, garam masala, mint, salt and plenty of black pepper. Form the meat mixture into 20 balls or ovals, put them on a couple of plates, cover while you make the sauce and chill.

To make the sauce, heat the oil in a large non-stick saucepan or sauté pan and gently fry the onions, garlic and ginger for about 6–8 minutes or until softened and lightly browned, stirring regularly. Add a little water if they begin to stick. Sprinkle over the chilli powder and garam masala and cook for a few seconds more, stirring continuously.

Pour the passata into the pan and stir in the lamb stock. Season the sauce well with salt and ground black pepper and bring to a simmer. Cover the pan loosely with a lid and simmer gently for 15 minutes, stirring occasionally.

While the sauce is simmering, brown the meatballs. Spray or brush a large non-stick frying pan with oil and place over a medium heat. Cook the meatballs in two batches for 6–8 minutes, turning occasionally, or until well browned on all sides.

Remove the sauce from the heat and blitz with a stick blender until as smooth as possible. (If you don't have a stick blender, leave to cool for a few minutes then transfer to a food processor and blitz to a purée.)

Gently drop all the meatballs into the sauce and return to a simmer. Cook, uncovered, for a further 25 minutes or until the meatballs are tender and the sauce is thick, stirring regularly. Drizzle over the yoghurt just before serving.

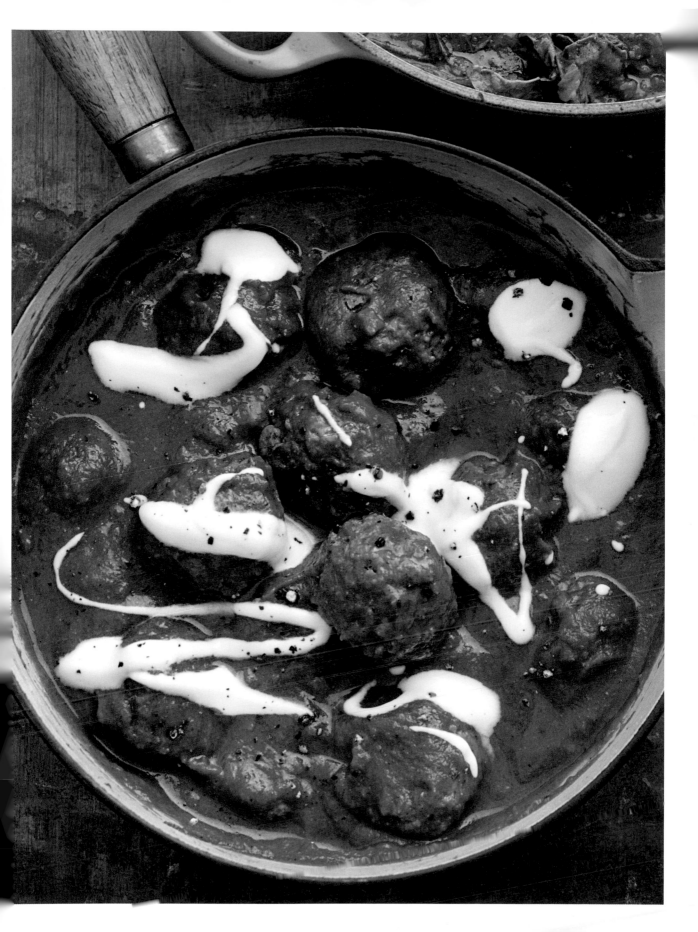

342

CALORIES
PER SERVING

simple beef madras

SERVES 6
PREP: 10 MINUTES
COOK: 1³/₄–2¹/₄ HOURS

1.2kg braising beef
    (ideally chuck steak)
1 tbsp sunflower oil
1 medium onion,
    finely chopped
2 garlic cloves, crushed
2 long red chillies,
    finely sliced
2 tbsp medium curry paste
1 tsp caster sugar
1 tsp flaked sea salt
2 x 400g cans chopped
    tomatoes
200ml beef stock (made
    with 1 beef stock cube)
thinly sliced red chilli,
    to garnish (optional)

Freeze the cooled curry
in a zip-seal bag or in
foil containers for up to
3 months. Thaw in the
fridge overnight. Reheat
thoroughly in a large, wide-
based saucepan, stirring
gently until piping hot.

Tip: You can also make
the curry with 12 boneless,
skinless chicken thighs and
leave out the stock. Cook
in the oven for just an hour
or until tender.

This is a hot beef curry that's very easy to make. Although it uses a ready-made curry paste, I like to add a couple of fresh chillies to give it a bit more zip. You can temper the spice with a cooling cucumber raita (see below).

Preheat the oven to 170°C/Fan 150°C/Gas 3. Remove any hard fat from the beef and cut into roughly 3cm chunks.

Heat the oil in a large flameproof casserole and fry the onion, garlic and red chillies over a high heat for 1 minute, while stirring. Add the curry paste and cook for a few seconds, stirring well.

Add the beef, sugar and salt and cook for 3 minutes, or until the beef is lightly coloured and well coated in the spice paste, turning regularly. Tip the tomatoes into the pan and stir in the beef stock.

Bring to a simmer, then cover with a lid and transfer the casserole carefully to the oven. Cook for 1¹/₂–2 hours or until the beef is beautifully tender and sauce has thickened. (If the sauce is still a little thin, return the casserole dish to the hob and simmer for 2–3 minutes, stirring regularly.) Garnish with sliced red chillies before serving if you like.

Cooling cucumber raita: Cut ¹/₂ cucumber into small chunks, put the chunks in a small bowl and season with a little flaked sea salt. Stir in 150g fat-free natural yoghurt and then loosely fold in 4 heaped tablespoons of chopped fresh mint leaves. Leave to stand for 10 minutes before serving. This also tastes great with lamb meatballs, falafels and tandoori chicken pieces. Serves 6. Calories per serving: 18

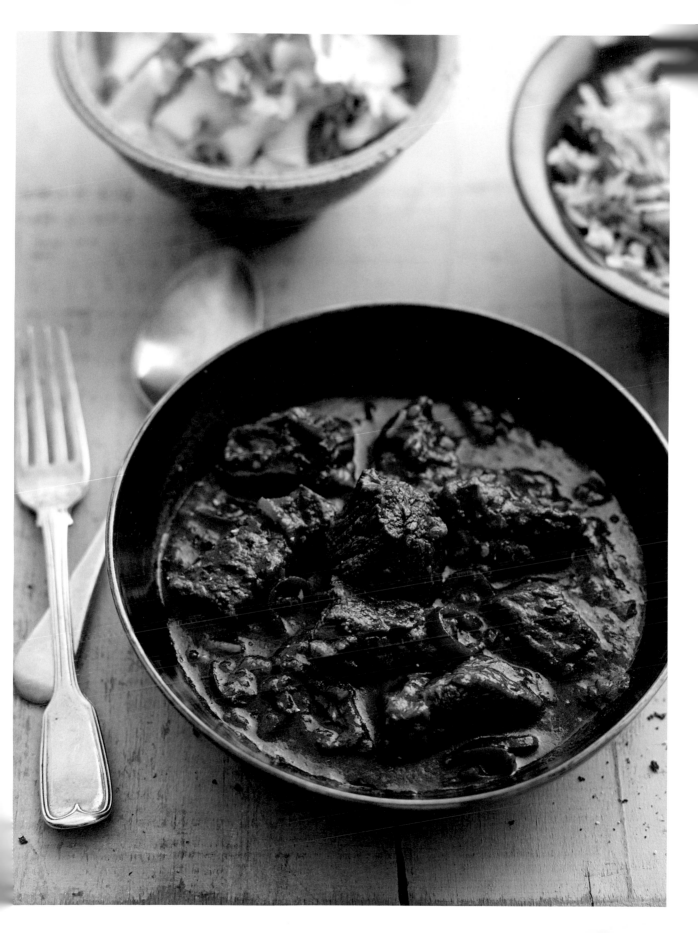

364
CALORIES
PER SERVING

pork vindaloo
with potatoes

SERVES 6
PREP: 15 MINUTES,
PLUS MARINATING TIME
COOK: 2–2¼ HOURS

1.2 kg pork leg steaks
    (boneless pork leg meat)
100ml red wine vinegar
2 tsp flaked sea salt, plus
    extra for seasoning
500ml cold water
2 bay leaves
650g potatoes, peeled
    and cut into roughly
    2.5cm chunks
1 long green chilli, very
    thinly sliced, to garnish
    (optional)

FOR THE CURRY PASTE
1 tbsp sunflower oil
2 medium onions,
    thinly sliced
6 garlic cloves,
    roughly chopped
6 red bird's eye chillies
    (do not deseed),
    roughly chopped
25g chunk fresh root
    ginger, peeled and
    roughly chopped
1 tbsp English mustard
    powder
2 tsp ground cumin
2 tsp ground coriander
1 heaped tsp paprika
    (not smoked)
1 tsp ground turmeric
1 tsp ground fenugreek
1 tsp ground cinnamon

This curry isn't frighteningly hot but is definitely a bit spicier than most of the curries here. Marinating the pork in vinegar helps tenderise the meat and marries very well with the spices. I use bird's eye chillies in this recipe but 3 long, red chillies and 1 teaspoon of hot chilli powder would work well too.

Trim the pork, discarding any fatty bits, and cut into roughly 4cm chunks. Put the vinegar and salt in a large non-metallic bowl. Add the pork and turn to coat it in the marinade. Cover and leave to marinate in the fridge for 2 hours.

While the pork is marinating, make the paste. Heat the oil in a large non-stick frying pan and cook the onions very gently over a medium-low heat for 15 minutes or until softened and lightly browned, stirring occasionally.

While the onions are cooking, put the garlic, chillies, ginger, mustard powder, cumin, coriander, paprika, turmeric, fenugreek and cinnamon in a food processor and blend to as fine a paste as possible. You may need to remove the lid and push the mixture down a couple of times with a spatula. If you don't have a food processor, pound the ingredients in a pestle and mortar instead.

Preheat the oven to 180°C/Fan 160°C/Gas 4. Tip the paste into the fried onions and cook together for 2 minutes, stirring regularly. Scrape everything into a large flameproof casserole dish. Drain the pork in a colander and reserve the marinade.

Add the pork to the spiced onions. Fry for 3–4 minutes or until the meat is coloured all over, turning regularly. Pour the reserved marinade and the water into the pan with the pork. Add the bay leaves and bring to a simmer. Cover the surface of the curry with a piece of baking parchment, then pop a lid on top. Cook in the oven for 45 minutes.

Take the casserole out of the oven and stir the potato chunks into the curry, cover with baking parchment and the lid and continue to cook for a further 50–60 minutes or until the pork and potatoes are very tender. Sprinkle with the sliced green chilli, if using, just before serving.

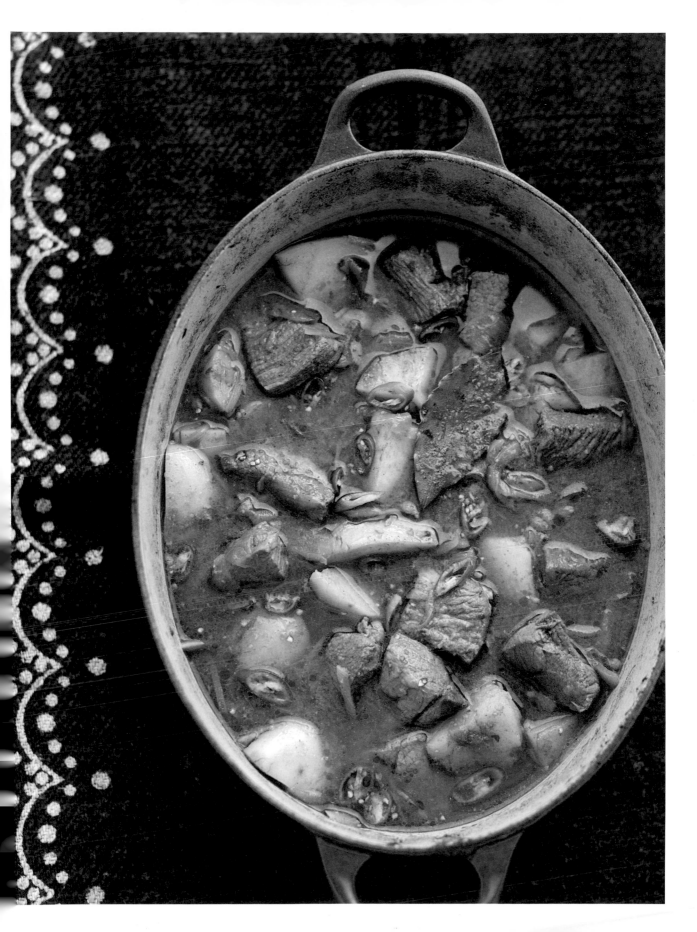

214

CALORIES
PER SERVING

king prawn balti

½ tbsp sunflower oil
2 tbsp medium or balti
   curry paste
½ medium onion,
   thinly sliced
1 tbsp mango chutney
4 ripe tomatoes, quartered
200ml cold water
200g peeled cooked king
   prawns, thawed if frozen
100g young spinach leaves

This curry is a classic takeaway staple that is very easy to replicate at home. Be sure to use curry paste rather than sauce as they produce very different results.

Heat the oil in a large non-stick frying pan or wok. Add the curry paste and onion and cook together over a medium heat for 3–4 minutes, stirring regularly, until the onion begins to soften.

Add the mango chutney, tomatoes and water, and increase the heat. Bring to a simmer. Leave to bubble for 5 minutes or until the tomatoes are soft but holding their shape and the liquid has reduced by half, stirring occasionally.

Scatter over the prawns and spinach leaves. Stir-fry for 2–3 minutes or until the prawns are heated through and the spinach has softened.

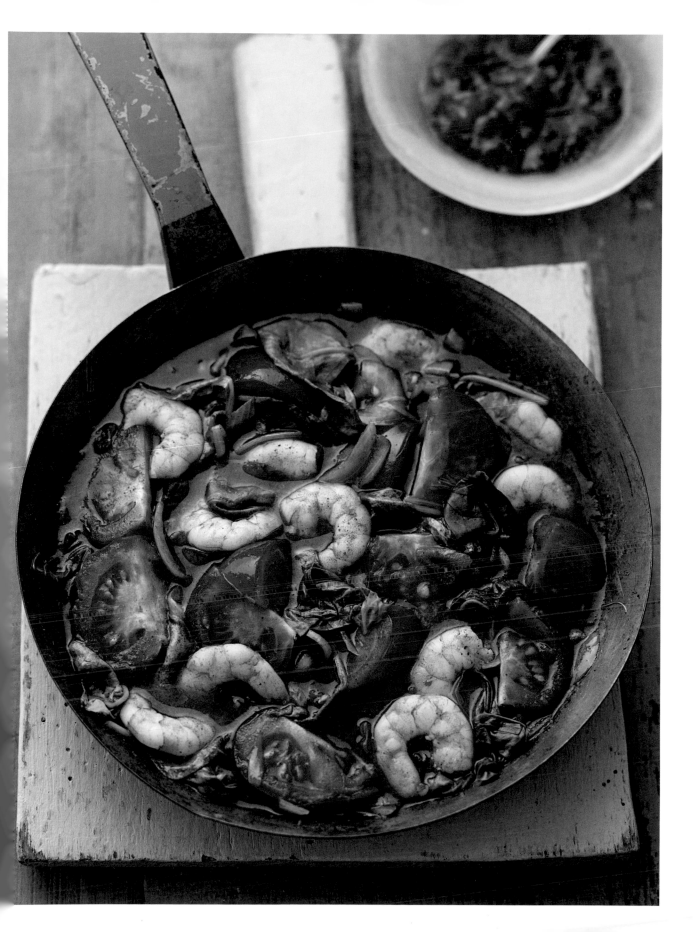

284
CALORIES
PER SERVING

vegetable biryani

SERVES 6
PREP: 15 MINUTES
COOK: 1¼ HOURS

½ cauliflower (around
300g), cut into small
florets
100g green beans, cut
into roughly 3cm lengths
2 carrots, cut into thin
diagonal slices
4 tsp sunflower oil
200g small chestnut
mushrooms, quartered
2 medium onions,
thinly sliced
2 tbsp medium curry paste
2 long green chillies,
finely chopped
4 garlic cloves, crushed
25g chunk fresh root ginger,
peeled and finely grated
1 tsp fine sea salt
400g can chopped
tomatoes
400ml cold water
3 fridge-cold eggs
20g fresh coriander,
roughly chopped

FOR THE RICE

500ml cold water
good pinch of saffron
200g basmati rice
8 cardamom pods,
lightly crushed
1 cinnamon stick,
broken in half
150g frozen peas

This biryani may look like a lot of work, but it makes a great family meal with no need to worry about side dishes. When topping the curry with the rice, be careful not to push it right to the edges or it will become too crunchy when baked.

Blanch the cauliflower, green beans and carrots in a large saucepan of boiling water for 3 minutes. Rinse under cold water, drain and set aside.

Heat half the oil in a large non-stick saucepan and fry the mushrooms over a high heat for 2–3 minutes or until golden brown, stirring regularly. Tip onto a plate and return the pan to the heat. Add 2 teaspoons more oil and the onions. Reduce the heat to medium-high and cook for 5 minutes or until golden.

Stir in the curry paste, chillies, garlic, ginger and salt. Cook for a minute, stirring constantly. Add the tomatoes and water. Bring to a gentle simmer and cook for 15 minutes, stirring occasionally. Preheat the oven to 190°C/Fan 170°C/Gas 5.

While the sauce is cooking, prepare the rice. Pour the cold water into a medium saucepan, add the saffron and bring to the boil. Add the rice, cardamom pods and cinnamon stick. Return to the boil and cook for exactly 8 minutes, stirring occasionally, until almost tender. Remove from the heat, stir in the peas, drain in a sieve and toss with half the coriander.

Spoon the cooked vegetable curry into a large, shallow ovenproof dish or flameproof casserole. Top with the rice, leaving a gap around the edge of the dish. Cover tightly with lightly oiled foil and cook in the oven for 45 minutes or until the rice is tender and steaming hot.

About 15 minutes before the biryani is ready, cook the eggs in boiling water for 9 minutes, then drain under running water until they are cool enough to handle. Peel the eggs and cut them into quarters.

Take the foil off the biryani and scatter the warm eggs into the rice. Sprinkle with the rest of the coriander just before serving.

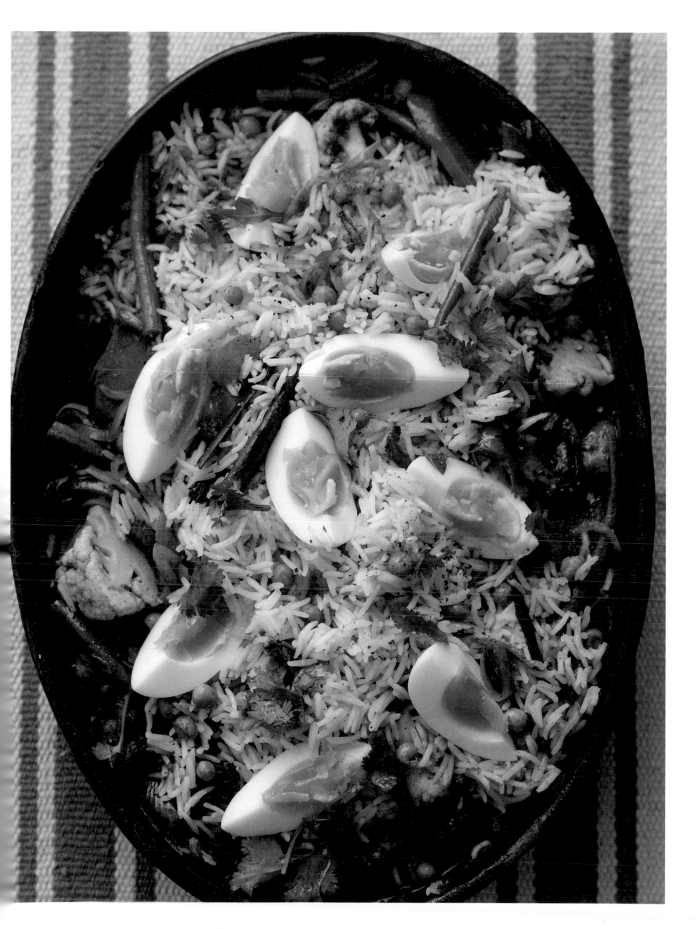

312
CALORIES
PER SERVING

mutter paneer

SERVES 4
PREP: 10 MINUTES
COOK: 25–30 MINUTES

1 tbsp sunflower oil
2 tsp cumin seeds
1 tsp black mustard seeds
2 medium onions, sliced
3 garlic cloves, thinly sliced
25g chunk fresh root ginger, peeled and finely grated
2 long green chillies, finely chopped (do not deseed)
2 tsp ground coriander
1 tsp ground turmeric
¼ tsp hot chilli powder
400g can chopped tomatoes
100ml fat-free natural yoghurt
½ tsp fine sea salt
oil, for spraying or brushing
225g paneer, drained and cut into roughly 1.5cm cubes
150g frozen peas
150ml cold water
ground black pepper

Freeze the cooled curry in a zip-seal bag or in foil containers for up to 3 months. Thaw in the fridge overnight. Reheat thoroughly in a large, wide-based saucepan, stirring gently until piping hot.

A hearty vegetarian curry made with peas and paneer (a mild Indian cooking cheese). You'll find paneer in larger supermarkets and Asian food stores. The richly spiced sauce is mellowed by the addition of yoghurt. The yoghurt may look a little grainy when it is first added to the sauce but will soon blend into the tomatoes as the liquid reduces.

Heat the oil in a large non-stick saucepan and fry the cumin and mustard seeds over a medium-high heat for a few seconds or until the seeds begin to crackle, stirring constantly. It's important that they don't burn or they will make the curry sauce taste bitter.

Add the onions, garlic, ginger and green chillies and cook for 5 minutes more, or until the onions are well softened, stirring. Sprinkle over the ground coriander, turmeric and chilli powder and cook for 1 minute, stirring continuously.

Tip the canned tomatoes into the pan, and add the yoghurt and salt. Season with lots of black pepper. Bring the sauce to a gentle simmer, stirring continuously. Cover the pan loosely with a lid and cook the sauce for 12–15 minutes or until thick. Don't let the sauce boil furiously and stir it regularly as it simmers, especially towards the end of the cooking time.

While the sauce is simmering, prepare the paneer. Place a small non-stick frying pan over a medium heat. Spray or brush with oil, then fry the paneer for about 5 minutes or until the cubes are lightly browned all over, turning regularly.

When the curry sauce is ready, stir in the frozen peas and 150ml cold water to loosen the sauce. Cook for a further 2–3 minutes or until hot, adding a little extra water if needed, then add the paneer and heat through gently. Check the seasoning – you may want a little extra salt or pepper – then serve with boiled basmati rice, if you like.

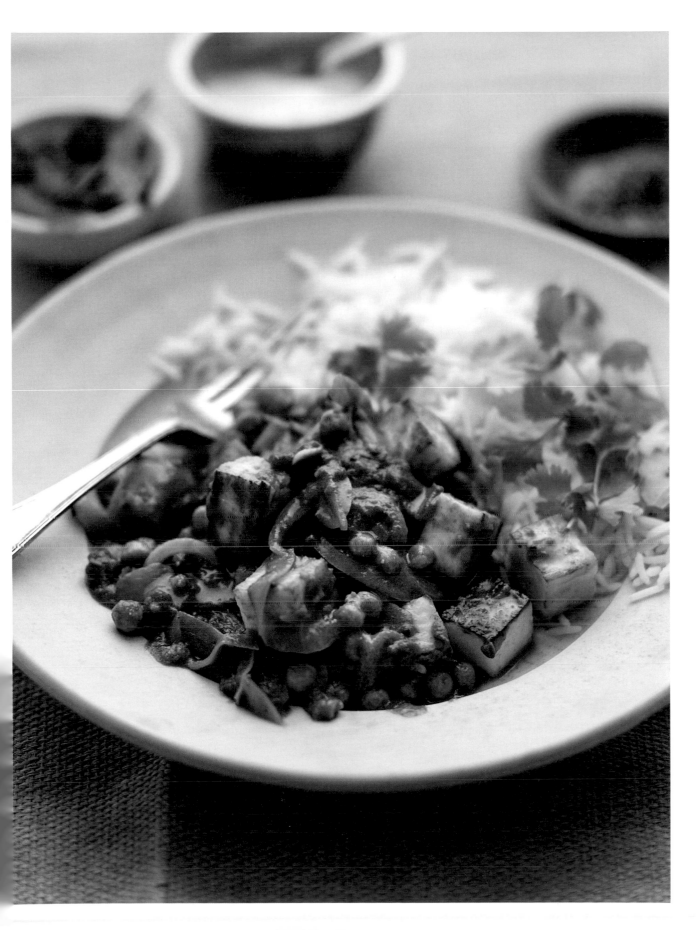

mixed vegetable dhal

SERVES 4
PREP: 10 MINUTES
COOK: 1¼–1¾ HOURS

200g yellow split peas, rinsed and drained
1.1 litres cold water
½ onion, thinly sliced
3 garlic cloves, crushed
20g chunk root ginger, peeled and finely grated
2 long green chillies, finely chopped
½ tsp ground turmeric
1 tsp fine sea salt, plus extra for seasoning
1 tbsp fresh lemon juice

FOR THE TOPPING
2 tsp sunflower oil
1 large onion, cut into thin wedges
1 yellow pepper, deseeded and cut into 3cm chunks
½ tsp black mustard seeds
½ tsp cumin seeds
1 tsp garam masala or medium curry powder
1 long green chilli, deseeded and finely sliced
4 medium tomatoes, quartered
fat-free natural yoghurt, to serve

Freeze the cooled curry without the topping in a zip-seal bag or freezer-proof containers for up to 3 months. Defrost in the fridge overnight. Reheat thoroughly in a large, wide-based saucepan, stirring regularly until piping hot and adding extra water if needed.

A veggie takeaway favourite, dhal can be very calorific because of the drenching of spiced oil and onions added at the end. My version has a mixture of lightly fried vegetables and chillies that add flavour and colour to the dish.

Tip the split peas into a large, heavy-based saucepan or flameproof casserole and cover with the water. Bring to the boil over a high heat. Skim off any foam that rises to the surface. Stir in the onion, garlic, ginger, chillies and turmeric.

Reduce the heat to low. Cover loosely with a lid and leave to simmer gently for 60–90 minutes or until the split peas are very tender and thick. It should have the texture of a thick soup. Stir fairly regularly, especially towards the end, and add a splash of water if it thickens too much before the split peas are tender.

When the dhal is ready, remove from the heat and season with salt and lemon juice to taste. Keep warm.

To make the topping, place a small frying pan over a medium-high heat and add the oil. Fry the onion and pepper for 5 minutes or until beginning to soften and lightly colour.

Stir the mustard seeds, cumin seeds, garam masala or curry powder, and chillies into the frying pan and cook for 2 minutes, stirring regularly. You may need to turn on your extractor fan or open a window as the chilli can make you cough.

Add the tomatoes and cook for 2–3 minutes more or until the vegetables are tender but still holding their shape. Spoon the spiced vegetables over the dhal. Serve with fat-free natural yoghurt (8 calories per tablespoon) if you like.

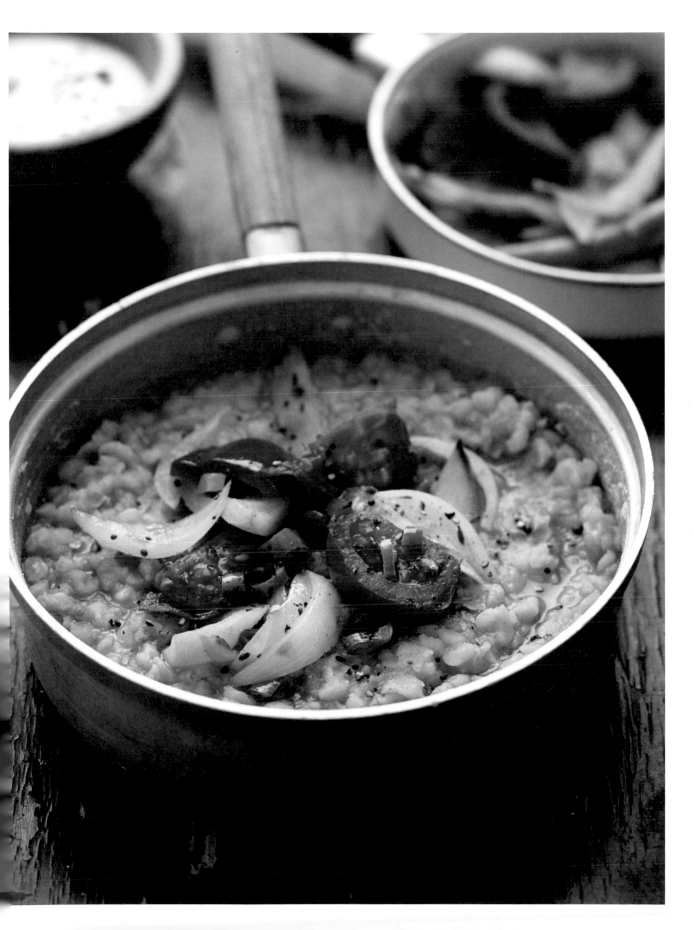

216
CALORIES
PER SERVING

channa masala

SERVES 4
PREP: 15 MINUTES
COOK: 1–1¼ HOURS

1 tbsp sunflower oil
2 onions, thinly sliced
4 garlic cloves, crushed
25g chunk fresh root ginger,
    peeled and finely grated
1 long green chilli, finely
    chopped (deseed first
    if you like)
1 tsp cumin seeds
1 tbsp ground coriander
2 tsp garam masala
2 heaped tsp paprika
    (not smoked)
2 tsp ground cumin
1 tsp ground turmeric
½ tsp hot chilli powder
400g can chopped tomatoes
½ tsp flaked sea salt,
    plus extra to season
1 tsp caster sugar
600ml cold water
2 x 400g can chickpeas,
    drained and rinsed
1 tbsp fresh lemon juice
20g fresh coriander,
    leaves roughly chopped,
    plus extra to garnish
ground black pepper
minted yoghurt (see
    page 40), to serve

Freeze the cooled curry
in a zip-seal bag or in foil
containers for up to 3 months.
Thaw in the fridge overnight.
Reheat thoroughly in a large,
wide-based saucepan, stirring
gently until piping hot.

This is one of my favourite veggie curries and is a fantastic dish even if you are a committed meat-eater. Add a little extra sugar if your tomatoes are particularly acidic and don't be tempted to cut the cooking time – it makes all the difference to the tenderness of the chickpeas. You can also serve this as an accompaniment – this quantity will make 6 servings of 144 calories.

Heat the oil in a large, wide-based non-stick saucepan or sauté pan. Add the onions, cover and fry over a low heat for 5 minutes, or until softened, stirring occasionally. Remove the lid, increase the heat a little and cook for 2 minutes more or until lightly browned, while stirring.

Stir the garlic, ginger, chilli and cumin seeds into the pan and fry together for 2 minutes, stirring continuously. Sprinkle over the ground coriander, garam masala, paprika, ground cumin, turmeric and chilli powder. Stir over a low heat for 2 minutes without burning. If the spices begin to stick, add a splash of cold water and continue cooking.

Tip the tomatoes into the pan and stir in the salt and sugar and 100ml of the water. Bring to the boil and cook for 4–5 minutes, while stirring, or until the sauce is very thick.

Add the chickpeas and the remaining water. Reduce the heat, so the sauce simmers gently. Cover loosely with a lid and cook for 45–55 minutes, or until the chickpeas are very tender and the sauce is thick, stirring regularly. If the sauce becomes too thick before the time is up, add a little more water.

Season the curry with salt and pepper and add the lemon juice to taste. Continue to cook for 2 minutes more. Stir in the chopped coriander and serve topped with a dribble of minted yoghurt (see page 40) and a few coriander leaves. Offer the rest of the yoghurt alongside.

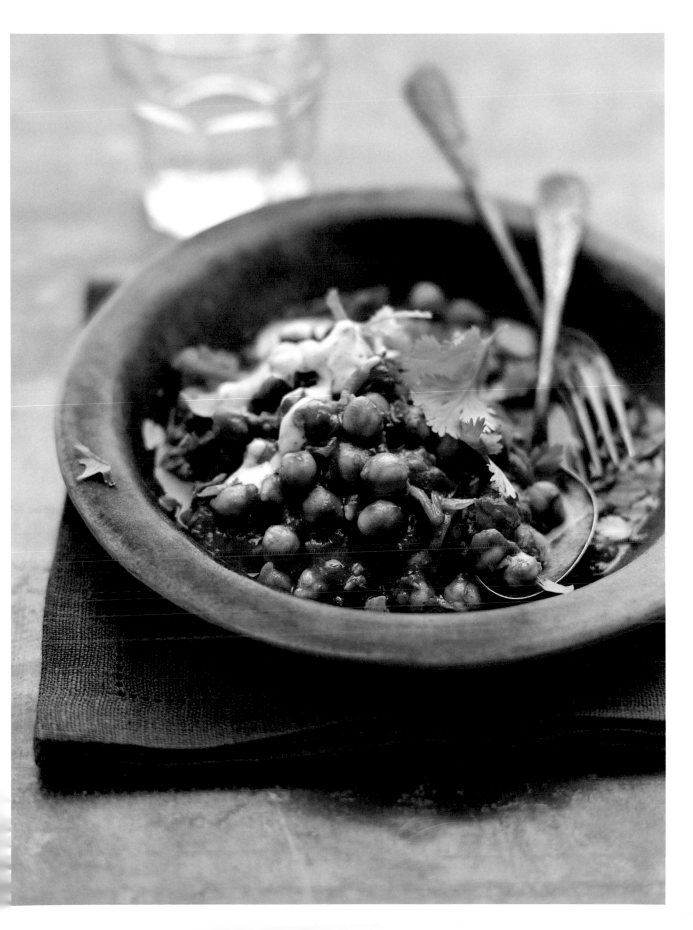

189
CALORIES
PER SERVING

light saag aloo

SERVES 4
PREP: 15–20 MINUTES
COOK: 25–30 MINUTES

3 potatoes (about 600g),
   peeled and cut into
   roughly 3cm chunks
½ tsp fine sea salt, plus
   extra to season
200g spinach leaves
   (not baby leaf spinach)
1 tbsp sunflower oil
2 medium onions,
   thinly sliced
1 tsp black mustard seeds
2 tsp cumin seeds
4 garlic cloves, finely sliced
15g chunk of fresh root
   ginger, peeled and
   finely chopped
1 long green chilli,
   finely chopped
   (deseed if you like)
2 tsp garam masala
½ tsp hot chilli powder
½ tsp ground turmeric
2–3 medium-large ripe
   tomatoes (about 200g),
   chopped into chunky
   pieces
200ml cold water
ground black pepper

Saag aloo is a popular restaurant and takeaway dish made with spiced potatoes and spinach. It's usually made with lots of oil, but I've created this one using just 1 tablespoon (and it tastes just as good!). I also like to use proper leafy spinach rather than the baby spinach that you can buy in bags as it has more depth of flavour – it's fine to use the other kind if you can't get hold of any.

Put the potatoes in a large saucepan and cover with cold water. Add the salt and bring to the boil. Reduce the heat slightly and simmer for 6–8 minutes or until the potatoes are tender, but still holding their shape. Drain in a colander. While the potatoes are cooking, wash the spinach and strip away any tough stalks. Roughly shred the leaves and put to one side.

Heat the oil in a large, deep non-stick frying pan or sauté pan and add the onions, mustard and cumin seeds. Cook for about 5 minutes over a medium heat or until the onions are softened, stirring regularly. Increase the heat and cook for a further 2–3 minutes or until the onions are nicely browned, stirring continuously.

Add the garlic, ginger, green chilli, garam masala, chilli powder, turmeric and spinach leaves. You'll need to add the spinach in 3–4 batches, allowing it to wilt and soften between each addition or you may have trouble fitting it in your pan. Fry for 1–2 minutes more, stirring well. Tip the tomatoes into the pan and add the potatoes and the water.

Bring to a simmer and cook for 5–6 minutes, or until the tomatoes are well softened, the potatoes are piping hot and almost all the liquid has evaporated, stirring regularly. Check the seasoning, adding more salt and ground black pepper if needed.

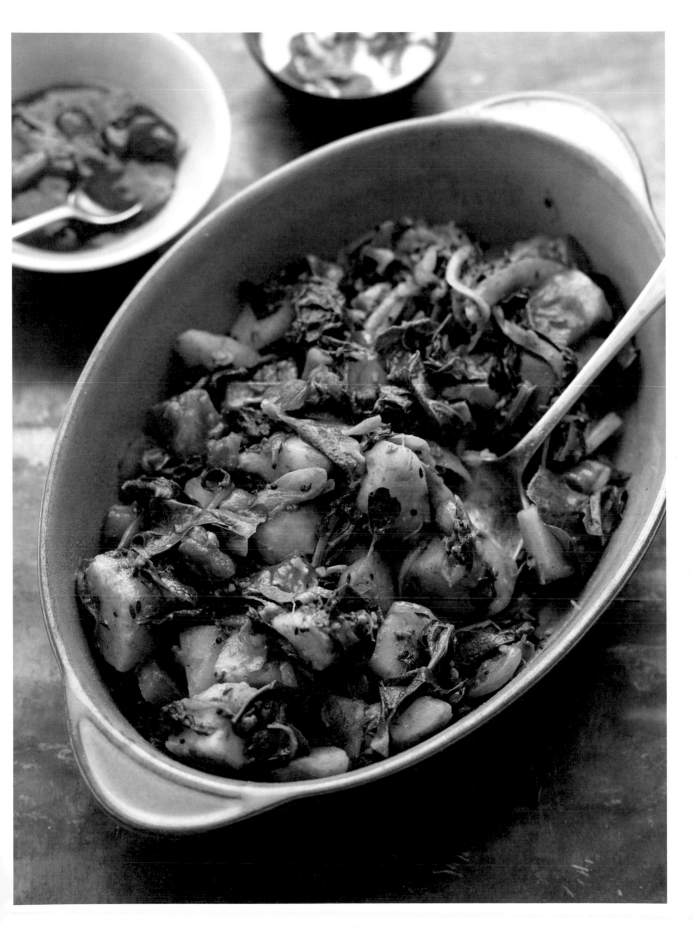

74
CALORIES
PER SERVING

masala poppadums with tomato and onion salad

SERVES 4
PREP: 10 MINUTES,
PLUS SOAKING TIME
COOK: 6–8 MINUTES

ready-to-cook poppadums,
    from a packet
1 tsp sunflower oil

FOR THE TOMATO
AND ONION SALAD
½ small onion, thinly sliced
1 tsp flaked sea salt
2 ripe tomatoes,
    roughly chopped
½ green or red chilli,
    finely diced (optional)
15g fresh coriander, leaves
    roughly chopped

Tip: Poppadums from an
Indian restaurant are larger
than the ready-to-cook
variety from the supermarket,
which is what you need for
this recipe. Watch your
poppadums carefully as
they are quick to burn if
cooked for too long.

Cooking poppadums in the microwave was a revelation to me. Just follow the packet instructions for ready-to-cook poppadums and, whatever you do, don't fry them. Brushed with only a tiny splash of oil, they contain 34 calories each. Alternatively, you could buy the ready-to-eat kind, bearing in mind they will bring around 43 calories each to the table. They are a great way to top up on your essential extra 300 calories too.

Put the onion in a bowl and toss with the salt. Leave to stand for 30 minutes. Cook the poppadums one at a time in a microwave oven, brushed with a little of the oil, according to the packet instructions.

Tip the onion into a sieve and rinse under cold running water – this will help remove any bitterness. Drain well and put the onion in a serving bowl.

Toss the onion with the tomatoes, chilli, if using, and chopped coriander leaves. Serve with the poppadums and minted yoghurt sauce (see below).

Minted yoghurt sauce: Mix 150ml fat-free natural yoghurt, 2 teaspoons prepared mint sauce (from a jar) and 1 teaspoon caster sugar in a serving bowl until well combined. Serves 4. Calories per serving: 27

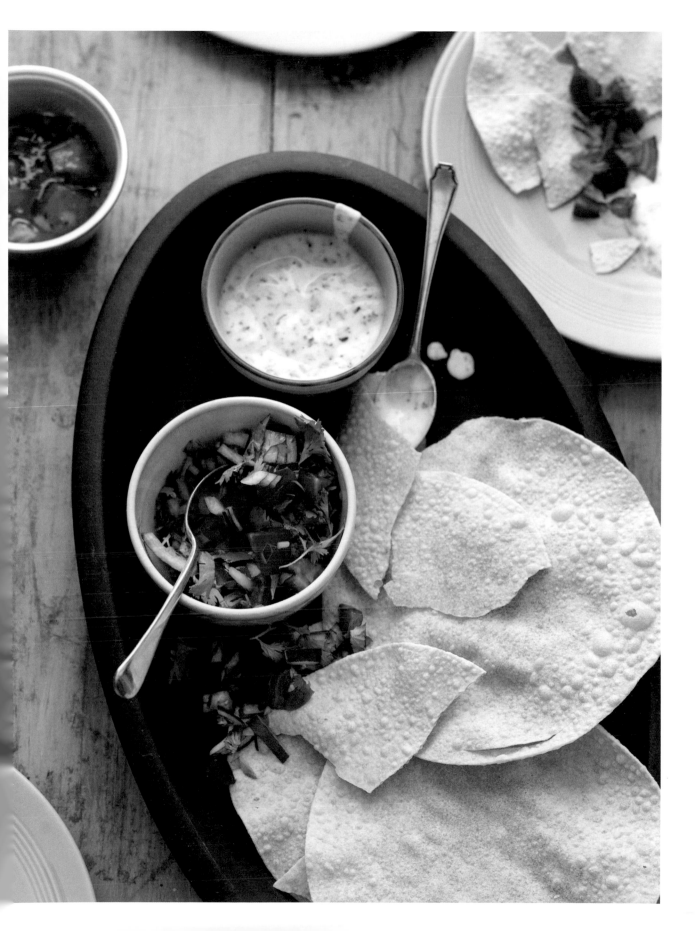

155
CALORIES
PER SERVING

skinny naan bread

SERVES 8
PREP: 20 MINUTES,
PLUS PROVING TIME
COOK: 3–5 MINUTES

300g plain flour, plus
    extra for rolling
3 tsp fast-action yeast
½ tsp bicarbonate of soda
1 tbsp caster sugar
1 heaped tsp fine sea salt
½ tsp nigella seeds (black
    onion seeds) (optional)
150ml lukewarm semi-
    skimmed milk
1 egg, beaten
oil, for greasing

Freeze naan breads in
a freezer bag for up to
1 month. Reheat from
frozen on a baking tray
in a moderate oven
before serving.

Tip: To make by hand,
put the dry ingredients in
a bowl, make a well in the
centre and add the milk
and egg. Mix together with
a pastry scraper or clean
hands until the dough starts
to come away from the
sides, then tip onto a lightly
floured surface and knead
for 10–15 minutes until soft
and pliable.

What would a curry be without some naan bread? I've tried to make this as light as possible, but do keep in mind that it is another starchy carbohydrate on top of rice. One or the other should be sufficient.

Put the flour, yeast, bicarbonate of soda, sugar, salt and nigella seeds (if using) in a food mixer fitted with a kneading paddle. With the motor running slowly, add the lukewarm milk and the beaten egg and mix together well. Increase the speed a little and knead the dough for 10 minutes or until soft and pliable with a lovely glossy surface.

Turn the dough out onto a floured surface, break into 8 portions and roll into balls. Taking a ball at a time, roll out on the floured surface into a teardrop shape with a slightly pointed end. The dough should be no more than 4mm thick.

Put the naans on a lightly oiled tea tray or large baking tray and cover loosely with oiled cling film. Leave in a warm place to prove for 45–60 minutes or until the dough is well risen.

Put a large baking tray in the oven and preheat to its hottest setting. This could be as high as 280°C/Fan 260°C/Gas 9, but don't worry if it is a little bit less. Pull the oven shelf out a little and place one of the naan breads quickly, but very carefully, on the preheated baking tray. Cook for about 2–2½ minutes or until the naan has puffed up and is lightly browned.

Place a large non-stick frying pan over a high heat. As soon as each naan bread is out of the oven, place it in the pan for about 5 seconds, until nicely toasted in places, then turn and do the same on the other side. Watch them very carefully as they will brown quickly.

Place the naan on a warmed serving dish or board. Cover with foil and a clean tea towel to keep warm and continue cooking the other naan breads in exactly the same way. Serve warm.

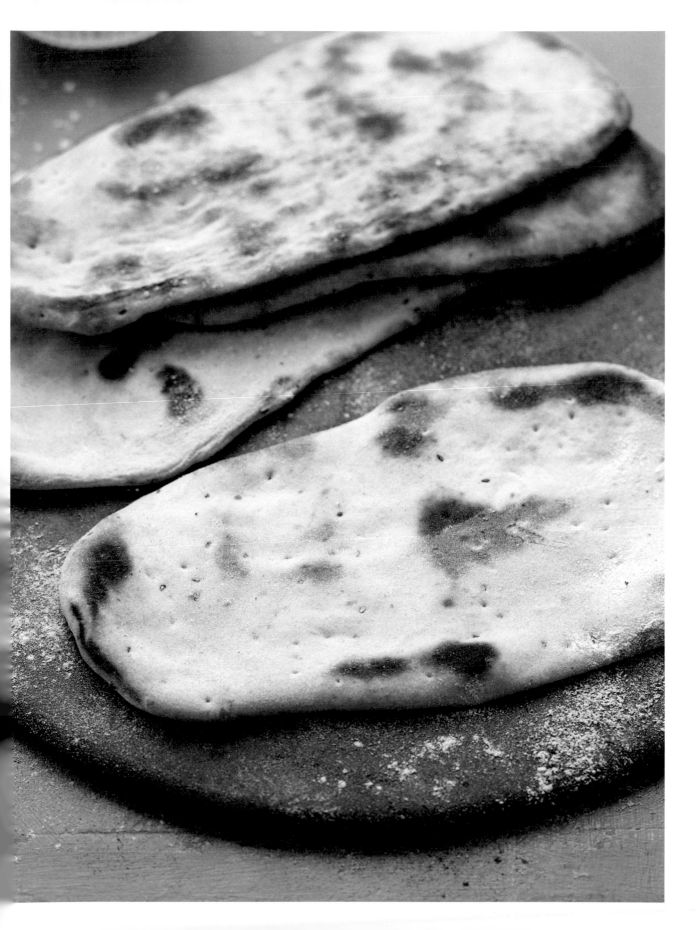

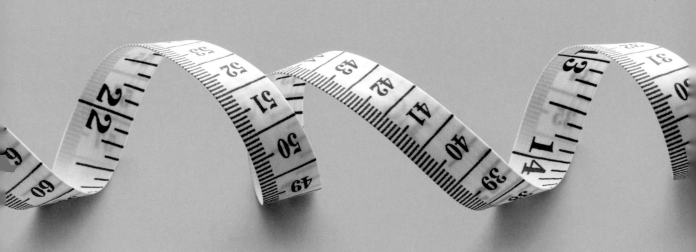

chinese

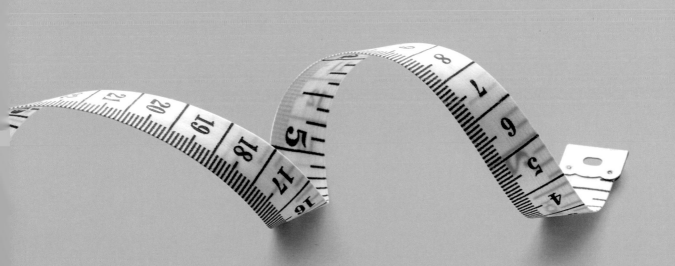

118
CALORIES
PER SERVING

sesame prawn toasts

SERVES 4

PREP: 15 MINUTES

COOK: 6–8 MINUTES

100g raw peeled prawns,
  thawed if frozen
2 spring onions, white
  part only, finely sliced
4 slices medium-cut
  white bread
2 tbsp sesame seeds
2 tbsp sunflower oil
flaked sea salt
ground white pepper
light or dark soy sauce
  and lime wedges,
  to serve

Open freeze the cooked
prawn toasts until solid then
wrap tightly in a freezer bag
for up to 1 month.

Tip: You can make an edible
garnish for the toasts by
soaking thin strips of spring
onion in iced water for
20 minutes until they curl.

Prawn toasts are a classic Chinese takeaway starter but they are usually deep-fried and soaked in fat. These triangles are made with just a little sunflower oil yet taste just as crispy. I initially tried to cut the calories by baking them, but these taste so much better and are still pretty low in cals.

Put the prawns and spring onions in a small food processor bowl. Season with a good pinch of salt and ground white pepper, then blend until almost smooth. You may need to remove the lid and push the mixture down a couple of times with a rubber spatula until the right consistency is reached.

Toast the bread on both sides until lightly browned. Put the toast on a large board, cut off the crusts and then cut diagonally in half. Spread each triangle thickly with the prawn paste, taking the mixture right up to the edges. Sprinkle evenly with sesame seeds and press down lightly so they stick to the paste.

Heat 1 tablespoon of the oil in a large non-stick frying pan and cook half the toasts prawn-side down over a medium heat for 2 minutes, or until the prawn topping is hot and completely pink and the sesame seeds are lightly toasted. Press gently with a spatula to help ensure every bit of the topping cooks.

Carefully turn the toasts over and cook on the other side for a further 1–2 minutes until hot throughout. Repeat with the remaining oil and toasts. Serve with soy sauce for dipping or drizzling and lime wedges for squeezing.

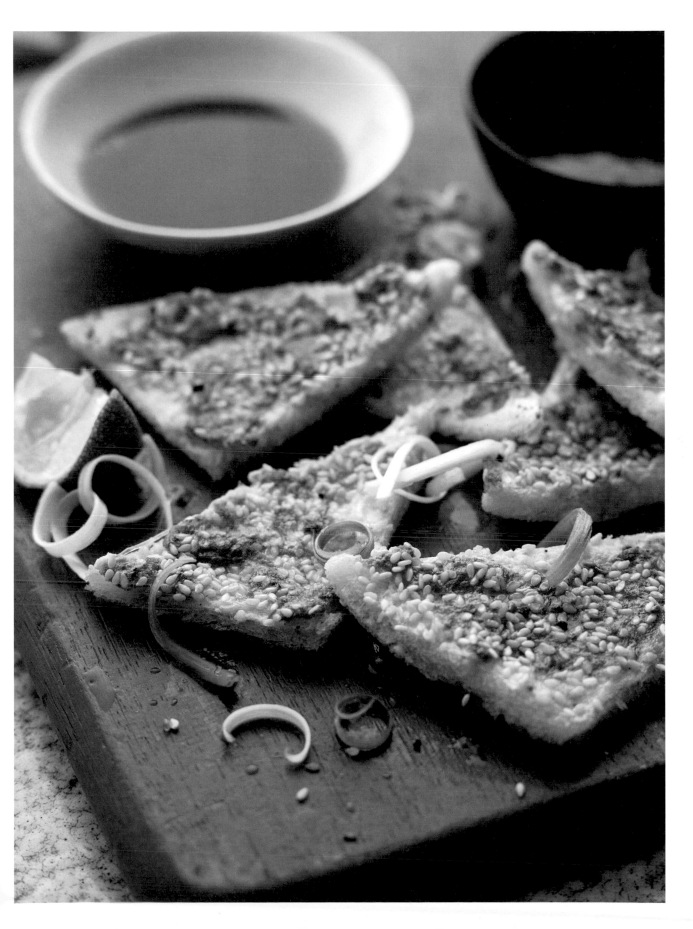

187
CALORIES
PER SERVING

vegetable spring rolls

SERVES 4

PREP: 15 MINUTES, PLUS COOLING TIME

COOK: 15 MINUTES

oil, for brushing or spraying

1 medium carrot, coarsely grated into long lengths

1 small red pepper, deseeded and cut into thin strips

3 garlic cloves, crushed

25g root ginger, peeled and finely grated

1 tsp soy sauce

100g bean sprouts, rinsed and drained

1 tsp cornflour

4 sheets filo pastry (each about 45g)

flaked sea salt

freshly ground black pepper

fresh coriander, to garnish

Vegetable filled spring rolls make an informal lunch or supper dish when served with a crunchy salad and dipping sauce. These rolls are lower in calories than usual as they are baked with only a light brushing of oil rather than deep fried.

Spray or brush a non-stick frying pan or wok with oil and place over a high heat. Add the carrot and pepper, garlic and ginger and stir-fry for 1 minute or until softened. Stir in the soy sauce and continue to cook for a further minute. Season with salt and pepper and then tip into a sieve over a bowl and leave to drain for 15 minutes. Once cool, mix in the bean sprouts and the cornflour.

Preheat the oven to 200°C/Fan 180°C/Gas 6. Cut each sheet of pastry into 3 long rectangles. Place one rectangle in front of you, with the short end closest, and brush or spray lightly with oil. Place roughly a twelfth of the cooled filling 5cm from the bottom and 2cm in from each side.

Fold up one side of the pastry and then fold over the ends. Roll up the pastry to encase the filling. Brush the outside of the pastry with a little more oil and place on a baking tray lined with baking parchment. Continue to make the remaining rolls in exactly the same way.

Bake for 10–15 minutes or until the pastry is golden and crisp. Serve warm with the dipping sauce (below) and fresh coriander to garnish.

Chilli and garlic dipping sauce: Mix 2 tablespoons caster sugar, 1 tablespoon white wine vinegar and 2 tablespoons water in a small saucepan. Add 1 finely sliced garlic clove and 1 finely sliced red bird's eye chilli. Warm through over a low heat for 1–2 minutes until the sugar dissolves, then leave to cool. Serves 4. Calories per serving: 30

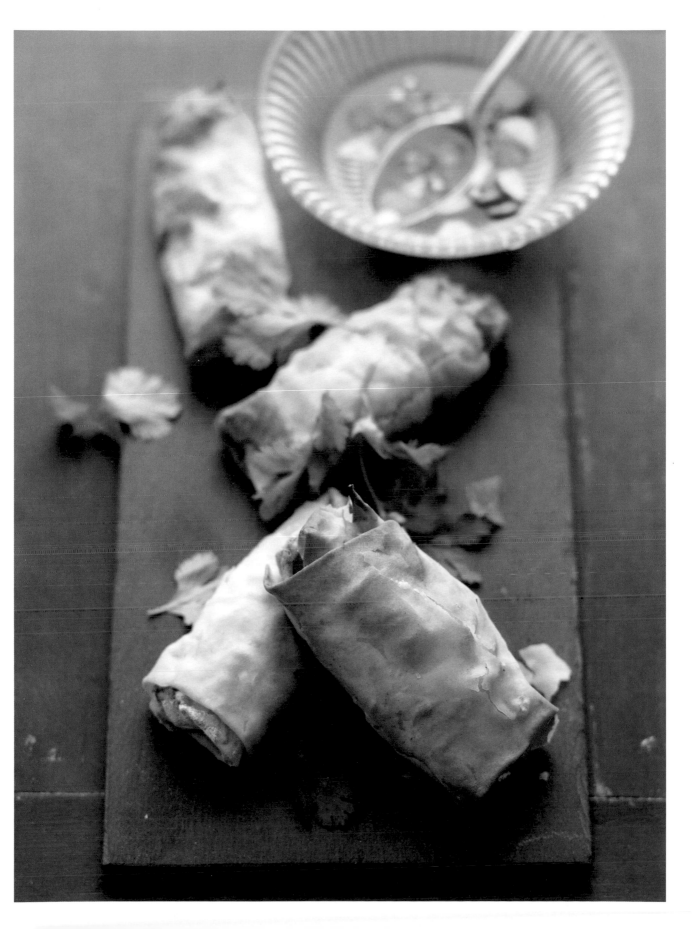

217
CALORIES
PER SERVING

shredded duck wraps
with hoisin sauce

SERVES 4
PREP: 10 MINS
COOK: 1 HOUR

2 duck leg quarters
2 tbsp dark soy sauce
1 tsp Chinese five-spice
   powder
3 spring onions
⅓ cucumber
2 little gem lettuce leaves
3 tbsp hoisin sauce

Tip: Using Chinese
pancakes instead of lettuce
will add around 33 calories
to each wrap.

Duck wraps are the perfect sharing starter or make a great light lunch. The nutritional calculation for this recipe includes the duck skin but you could save around 100 calories per serving if you do not have the skin.

Preheat the oven to 180°C/Fan 160°C/Gas 4. Rub the duck legs with the soy sauce and sprinkle over the five-spice powder evenly. Place on a rack over a baking tray lined with foil and bake for 50–60 minutes, or until the skin is crisp and dark golden brown.

Just before the duck is ready, prepare the vegetables. Trim the spring onions, cut in half and slice into very thin strips lengthways. Cut the cucumber into roughly 6cm long, thin matchsticks. Trim the lettuce and carefully separate the leaves. Wash and drain the leaves.

After baking, check the duck is tender using a fork. It should pull apart easily. Shred the duck by tearing it apart with 2 forks. Place the duck, cucumber, spring onions and sauce on a serving platter or board for sharing.

To eat, place a few strips of cucumber and spring onion on a lettuce leaf and add some warm, shredded duck. Spoon over a little hoisin sauce.

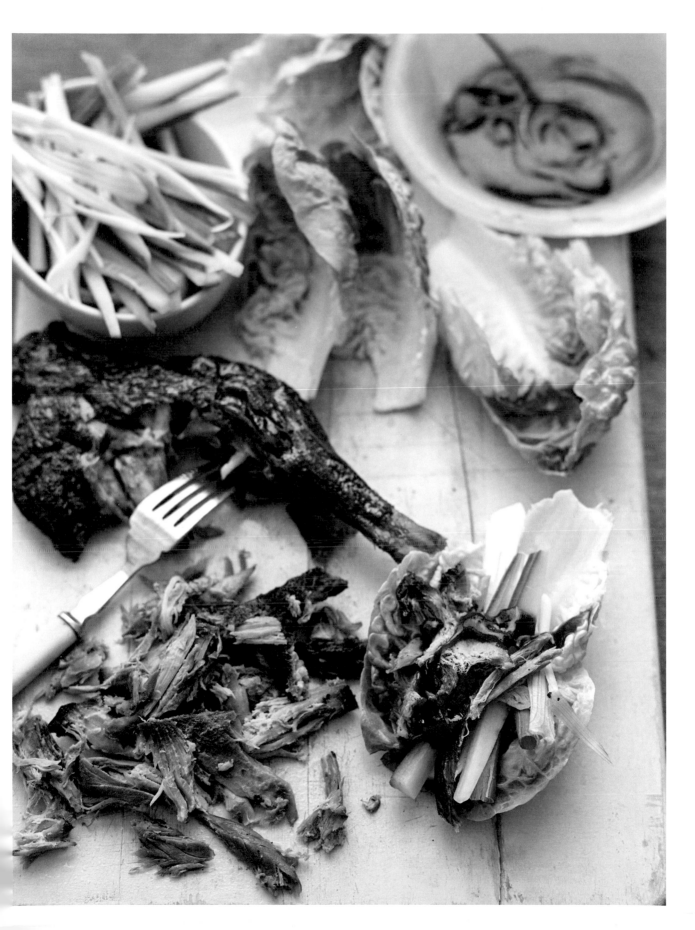

dim sum

SERVES 4

PREP: 25 MINUTES, PLUS STANDING TIME

COOK: 8–10 MINUTES

FOR THE PASTRY

300g strong white bread flour, plus extra for rolling

½ tsp fine salt

200ml just-boiled water

FOR THE FILLING

250g minced pork

15g chunk fresh root ginger, finely grated

2 garlic cloves, crushed

½ tsp flaked sea salt

½ tsp ground black pepper

2 spring onions, trimmed and finely sliced

½ tsp dried chilli flakes

1 tsp toasted sesame oil

soy sauce, to serve

Open freeze the uncooked dumplings until solid and layer with parchment in a freezer-proof container. Cook from frozen as above, but add a couple of extra minutes to the steaming time and ensure the filling is fully cooked before serving.

Fairly labour intensive, but these little dumplings are worth the effort and are fun to make too. They freeze beautifully, so you can make a big batch and keep some aside, ready to cook another time. The delicate pork and ginger flavour makes these a deliciously light supper when served with stir-fried vegetables or a salad.

To make the pastry, mix the flour, salt and water in a large heatproof bowl. When it is cool enough to handle, knead the dough really well for 10 minutes until very pliable. Wrap in cling film and leave to stand for 30 minutes.

Place the dough on a lightly floured work surface and knead for 5 minutes. Take one-third of the dough and roll it out very thinly, turning regularly – it should be only 2mm thick, so you can almost see the work surface through it. Cut out 8 circles with a 10cm circular pastry cutter, stacking the discs with a dusting of flour in between to stop them sticking. Take half the remaining dough and do the same. Continue until all the dough is used up.

Mix all the filling ingredients together in a large bowl. Take a pastry disc and place it in the palm of your hand. Put a teaspoonful of the filling in the centre and brush around the edge with a little cold water. Bring one side over the filling and fold into a half moon shape. Put to the side and make the other dumplings in exactly the same way.

Half fill a medium saucepan with water and bring to a simmer. Line a bamboo steamer with a disc of baking parchment and punch 15 small holes with the end of a skewer. Place over the simmering water. Arrange 6–8 dumplings inside the steamer. Cover with a lid and steam for about 10 minutes or until the filling is cooked and the dumpling pastry is tender. Cover the steamed dumplings with foil and place in a low oven to keep warm. Steam the rest of the dumplings in the same way. Serve the warm dumplings with a small bowl of soy sauce for dipping.

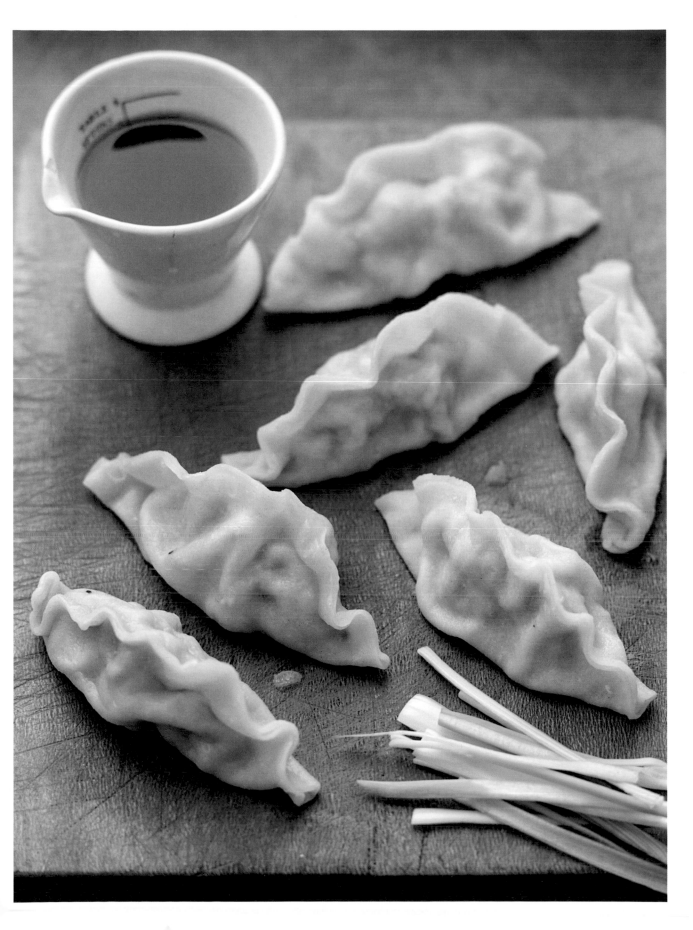

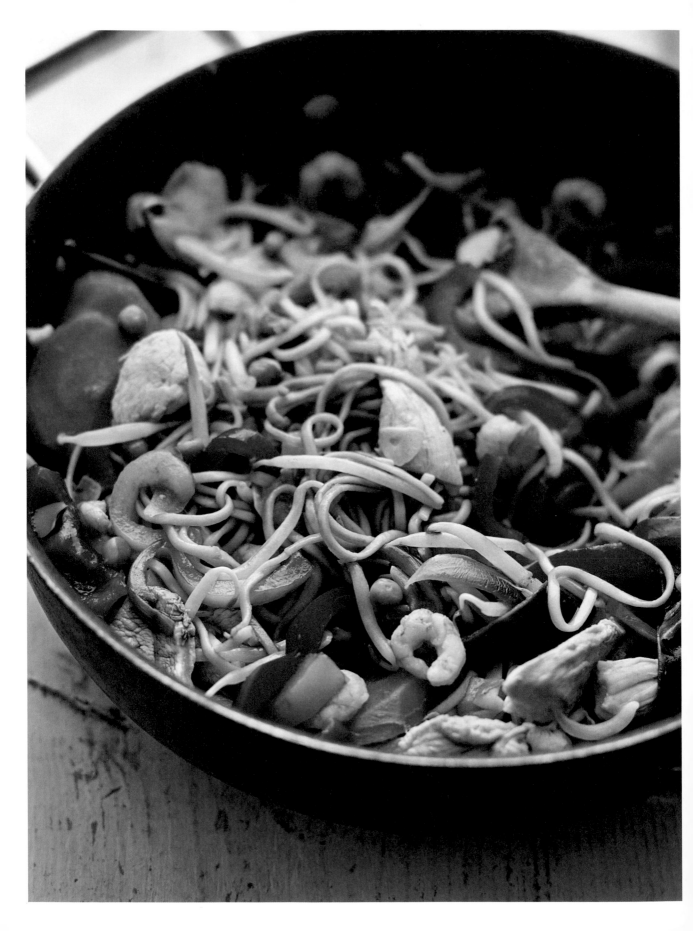

327

special chow mein

SERVES 4
PREP: 20 MINUTES
COOK: 10-12 MINUTES

100g dried medium
  egg noodles
1½ tsp sunflower oil
2 boneless, skinless chicken
  breasts, thinly sliced
1 medium red onion,
  cut into 12 wedges
1 red and 1 yellow pepper,
  deseeded and sliced
2 medium carrots,
  thinly sliced
2 tsp cornflour
1 tbsp light soft brown sugar
3 tbsp dark soy sauce
2 tbsp dry sherry or mirin
  (rice wine)
100ml cold water
150g cooked and peeled
  prawns, thawed if frozen
75g frozen peas
20g chunk fresh root ginger,
  peeled and finely grated
3 garlic cloves, very
  thinly sliced
100g bean sprouts,
  rinsed and drained
ground black pepper

Chow mein is usually very noodle heavy, but I've made mine with lots of colourful vegetables, plus lean chicken breast and prawns, rather than filling it up with carbs. I recommend you prepare all the vegetables and chicken before you start cooking, as the frying process only takes 10 minutes from start to finish.

Half fill a medium saucepan with water and bring to the boil. Add the noodles and cook for 3 minutes, or follow the packet instructions, until tender. Drain in a sieve under running water until cold and toss with ½ teaspoon of the oil. Set aside.

Heat the remaining oil in a large wok or deep, non-stick frying pan. Fry the chicken and onion over a high heat for 2-3 minutes or until they are beginning to lightly brown, turning regularly. Add the peppers and carrots and fry for 2 minutes more.

While the chicken and vegetables are frying, mix the cornflour and sugar together in a bowl and gradually stir in the soy sauce, sherry or mirin and the water. Put to one side.

Next, add the cooked noodles, prawns, peas, ginger and garlic to the pan. Grind some ground black pepper over the top and stir-fry together for 2-3 minutes or until the noodles, prawns and peas are hot. I use a couple of wooden spoons to toss the ingredients.

Give the soy mixture a good stir and pour it into the pan. Add the bean sprouts and toss everything together for 1-2 minutes or until piping hot and glossy.

134
CALORIES
PER SERVING

chicken and sweetcorn soup

SERVES 4

PREP: 5 MINUTES

COOK: 15 MINUTES

1 litre cold water

1 chicken stock cube

1 cooked, skinless chicken breast (about 125g), torn into thin strips

195g can sweetcorn, drained

6 spring onions, finely sliced

3 tbsp cornflour, mixed with 3 tbsp cold water

1 egg, beaten

It wasn't until I made Chinese-style chicken and sweetcorn soup for the first time that I realised its soft, silky texture comes from strands of beaten egg poached in the hot stock. It's warming on a cold, rainy day but also light enough to enjoy when the sun is shining.

Bring the cold water to the boil in a large saucepan. Add the stock cube and stir until dissolved.

Stir the chicken strips and sweetcorn into the stock and simmer gently for 5 minutes. Add the spring onions and the cornflour mixture and cook for a further 3–4 minutes, stirring continuously, until the stock thickens.

Remove the pan from the heat and pour the beaten egg into the soup. Stir just a couple of times with a fork, to swirl the egg into strands as it cooks in the hot stock.

Ladle the soup into small bowls and serve.

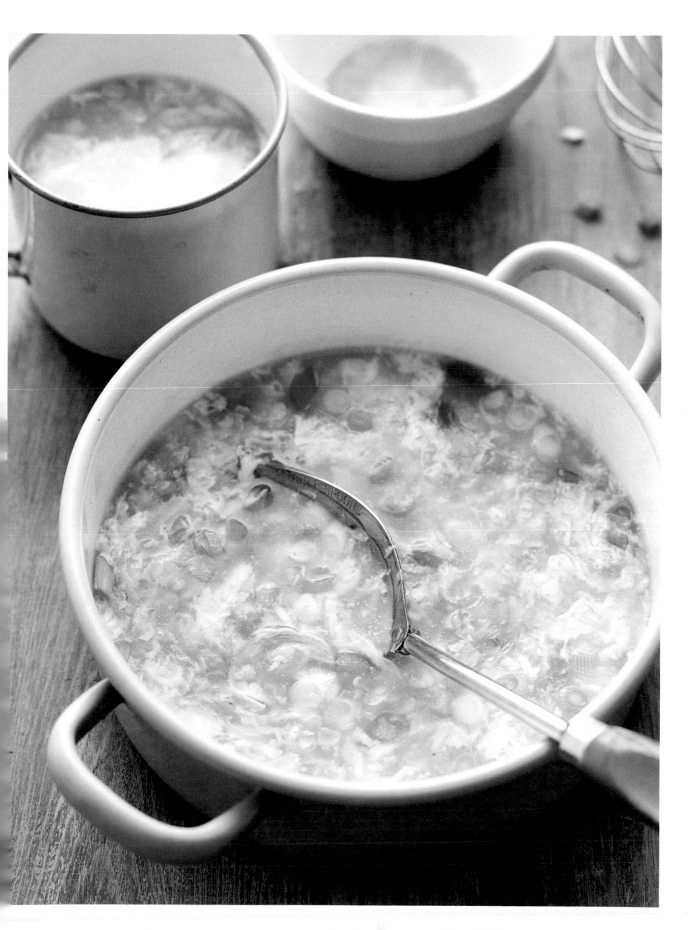

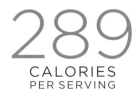

289
CALORIES
PER SERVING

kung pao chicken with broccoli

SERVES 4
**PREP: 20 MINUTES,
PLUS MARINATING TIME**
COOK: 10 MINUTES

3 boneless, skinless
  chicken breasts
2 tsp sunflower oil
250g small broccoli
  florets, halved if large
8 spring onions, cut into
  4cm lengths
2 garlic cloves, finely
  chopped
225g can water chestnuts,
  drained and halved
25g roasted salted peanuts
  or cashew nuts (or a
  mixture), roughly
  chopped
100ml cold water
2 tsp sesame oil

FOR THE MARINADE
1 tbsp cornflour
3 tbsp mirin (rice wine)
  or dry sherry
3 tbsp dark soy sauce
2 tsp white wine or
  Chinese rice vinegar
2 tbsp soft light
  brown sugar
1 tsp dried chilli flakes

I've added broccoli to my version of this dish as the tiny flower heads soak up the glossy sauce and hold the chopped nuts. I like to use roasted nuts – they have a golden colour and a good nutty flavour so you can get away with a minimal amount. Don't be tempted to add more as they are terrifically high in calories – about 150 calories per 25g.

Put the chicken breasts on a board and cut each one into roughly 2cm chunks. To make the marinade, put the cornflour in a large non-metallic bowl and stir in the mirin or sherry until smooth. Add the soy sauce, wine or vinegar, brown sugar and chilli flakes. Stir the chicken into the marinade until well coated, then cover and chill for at least 30 minutes and up to 1 hour.

Drain the chicken in a sieve over a bowl, turning to release as much of the liquid as possible into the bowl. Reserve the marinade.

Place a large non-stick frying pan or wok over a medium-high heat. Add the sunflower oil to the pan and as soon as it is hot, gently add the chicken and stir-fry for 3 minutes or until lightly coloured all over. Watch out when you add the chicken as it could spit. Scatter the broccoli florets into the pan with the chicken and stir-fry for a further 2 minutes.

Add the spring onions, garlic, water chestnuts and nuts to the pan and stir-fry for 2 minutes more. Pour the reserved marinade, water and the sesame oil over the chicken and vegetables and cook for 2 minutes or until the chicken is cooked, the broccoli is tender and the sauce is thickened and glossy, stirring as the sauce thickens.

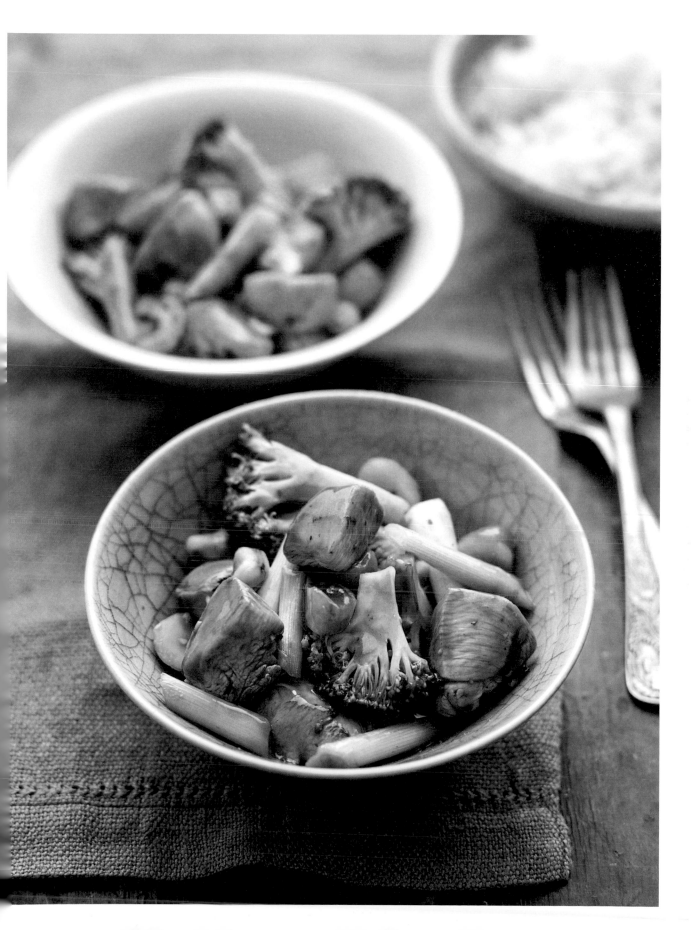

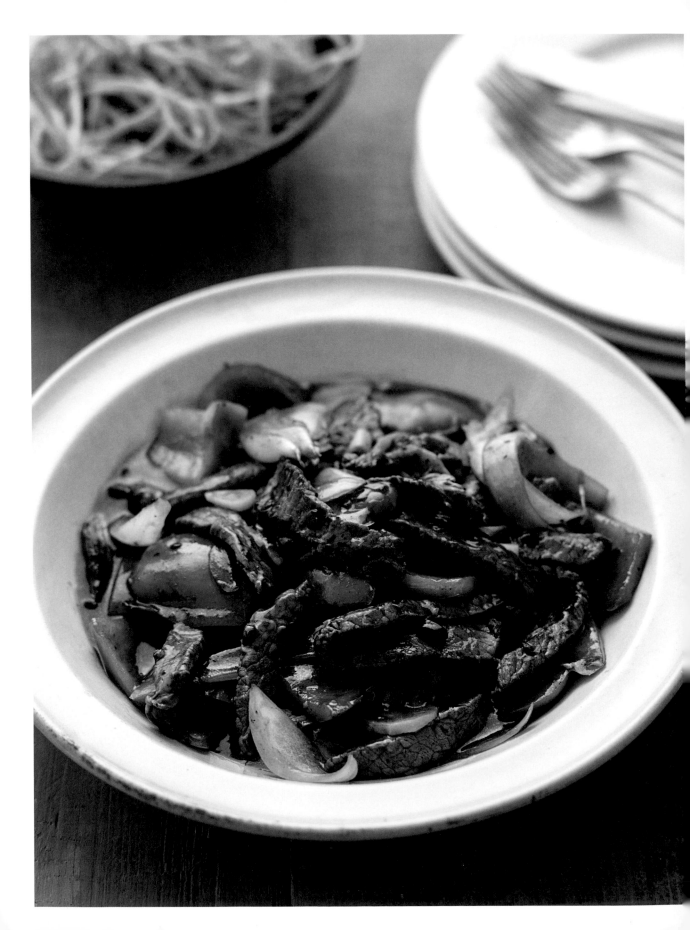

225

beef with green peppers in black bean sauce

SERVES 4
PREP: 15 MINUTES
COOK: 18–20 MINUTES

1 tbsp cornflour
2 tbsp mirin (rice wine)
   or dry sherry
120g sachet black
   bean sauce
100ml cold water
400g rump or sirloin steak
2–3 tsp sunflower oil
1 medium onion, cut into
   12 wedges
2 green peppers, deseeded
   and cut into 3cm chunks
2 garlic cloves, very thinly
   sliced
20g chunk fresh root
   ginger, peeled and
   very thinly sliced
flaked sea salt
ground black pepper

Tip: I've found black bean
sauce sachets milder than
jar sauces, but if using
sauce from a jar, add half
the sauce first then taste
and add more if needed.

A takeaway and restaurant classic, black bean sauce is made from fermented and salted soya beans, which gives it the characteristic salty, savoury flavour.

Mix the cornflour with the mirin or sherry in a small bowl until smooth, then stir in the black bean sauce and water. Put to one side. Trim the beef of all hard fat and cut into 5cm-wide strips. Season the beef well with a little salt and lots of black pepper.

Heat 1 teaspoon of the oil in a large non-stick frying pan or wok over a high heat and stir-fry the beef in two batches until well browned, adding a tiny splash more oil between batches if needed. Each batch will take about 3 minutes over a high heat. Transfer the beef to a plate each time a batch is ready.

Return the pan to the heat, add another teaspoon of oil and stir-fry the onion and peppers for 4 minutes, or until well softened and lightly coloured, then add the garlic and ginger and cook for 1 minute more.

Return the meat to the pan, pour over the reserved sauce and stir-fry together for 2–3 minutes or until the beef is hot and glossy.

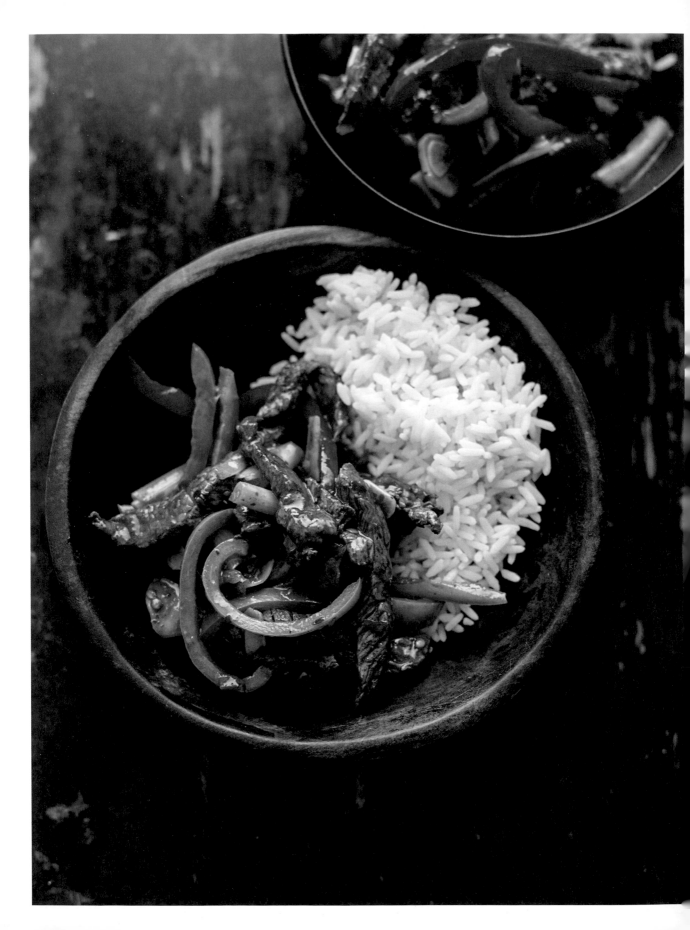

217
CALORIES
PER SERVING

chilli beef stir-fry

SERVES 4
PREP: 15 MINUTES
COOK: 15 MINUTES

400g thin-cut beef
frying steak
½ tsp Chinese five-spice
powder
1 tbsp cornflour
2 tbsp mirin (rice wine)
or dry sherry
2 tbsp white wine vinegar
2 tbsp dark soy sauce
2 tbsp tomato ketchup
2 tbsp crushed chilli paste
(from a jar)
150ml water
1 tbsp sunflower oil,
plus 1 tsp
1 red and 1 green
pepper, deseeded
and thinly sliced
2 garlic cloves,
very thinly sliced
20g chunk fresh root ginger,
peeled and thinly sliced
6 spring onions, trimmed
and cut into 2cm slices

A really fiery stir-fry. Serve with your choice of vegetables and perhaps a small portion of rice or noodles (see essential extras on page 180). It's worthwhile having all of your ingredients ready to go before you start as it cooks quickly.

Trim the beef of all hard fat and sinew and cut into thin strips. Put it in a bowl and toss with the five-spice powder. Mix the cornflour with the mirin or sherry in a separate bowl until smooth and stir in the vinegar, soy sauce, ketchup, crushed chilli and water and put to one side.

Heat the oil in a large non-stick frying pan or wok over a high heat and stir-fry the beef in three batches until well browned, adding 1 teaspoon oil in between batches if needed. Each batch will take about 3 minutes. Put the beef on a plate each time a batch is cooked.

Return the pan to the heat and stir-fry the peppers for 2 minutes, then add the garlic, ginger and spring onions and cook for 1 minute more.

Return the meat to the pan, pour over the reserved sauce and stir-fry together for 2–3 minutes or until the beef is hot and glossy.

284
CALORIES
PER SERVING

sweet and sour pork

SERVES 4

PREP: 20 MINUTES

COOK: 10–12 MINUTES

500g pork tenderloin (fillet)
oil, for spraying or brushing
1 medium red onion,
    cut into 12 wedges
1 red and 1 green pepper,
    deseeded and cut into
    roughly 3cm chunks
6 spring onions,
    diagonally sliced
flaked sea salt
ground black pepper

**FOR THE SWEET
AND SOUR SAUCE**

435g can pineapple
    chunks in juice
2 garlic cloves, crushed
20g chunk fresh root
    ginger, peeled and cut
    into thin matchsticks
2 tbsp dark soy sauce
2 tbsp white wine vinegar
2 tbsp caster sugar
2 tbsp tomato ketchup
$\frac{1}{2}$ tsp dried chilli flakes
1 tbsp cornflour
1 tbsp cold water

**This pork stir-fry isn't swamped with the usual over-sweet
and cloying sauce but is just lightly coated with a hint of
chilli heat. It's colourful and very filling but you can always
add a small portion of rice or noodles.**

To make the sauce, drain the pineapple chunks in a sieve
and reserve the juice in a bowl. Set the pineapple chunks
aside and stir the garlic, ginger, soy sauce, vinegar, sugar,
ketchup and chilli flakes into the juice until thoroughly
combined. Set aside.

Trim the pork of any visible fat and sinew, then cut into 1.5cm
slices and season with salt and lots of black pepper. Spray or
brush a large non-stick wok or frying pan with oil and stir-fry
the onion and peppers for 3 minutes over a high heat. Tip into
a bowl.

Brush or spray the pan with more oil and add the pork. Fry
for 3 minutes, or until lightly browned on both sides, turning
the slices every now and then. Stir in the onion, peppers and
pineapple pieces. Cook together for 2 minutes, while stirring.

Add the sweet and sour sauce to the pan and bring to a simmer
over a medium heat. Cook for 1 minute, stirring regularly, or
until the pork is cooked through. Mix the cornflour and cold
water until smooth and add to the pork and vegetables along
with the spring onions. Cook for 1 minute more or until the
sauce is thickened and glossy, stirring continuously.

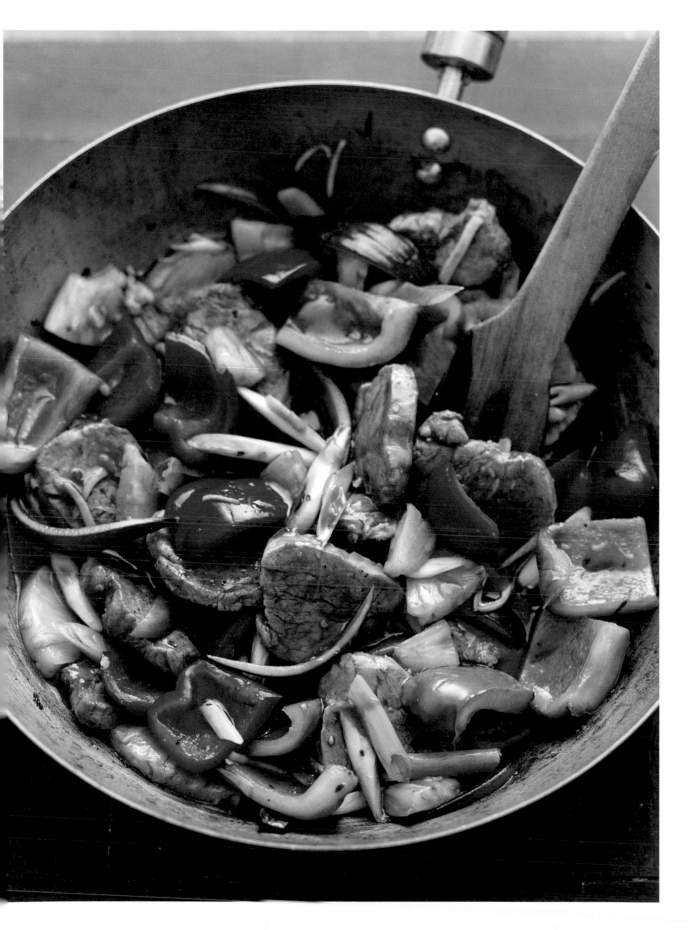

salt and pepper squid

SERVES 4
PREP: 20 MINUTES
COOK: 2–3 MINUTES

300g cleaned squid cones
1 tbsp black peppercorns
1 tsp dried chilli flakes
1 tbsp flaked sea salt
1 tsp plain flour
2 tsp sunflower oil
lime wedges, for squeezing
chilli dipping sauce
   (see right), to serve

Tip: It's important not to overcook the squid as it will toughen quickly; as soon as it is turns from translucent to opaque and curls up at the edges, it is ready.

This may not have a crispy batter but it has more than enough flavour. You can use either black peppercorns alone or a mixture of 2 teaspoons black peppercorns and 1 teaspoon Sichuan peppercorns for a more tingly effect. Serve with chilli dipping sauce (see below) as a starter or with drinks instead of nuts or crisps.

Cut the squid cones up the side, open out and scrape the membranes away from the side. Pat lightly with kitchen paper. Score the inside of each cone in a roughly 1cm criss-cross pattern with the tip of a knife, working diagonally across the flesh. Next, cut the squid into wide strips – cutting into strips rather than rings means it will fry into lovely scoop shapes that are ideal for dipping.

Tip the peppercorns, chilli flakes and salt into a pestle and mortar and pound hard until roughly the texture of coarsely ground black pepper. Transfer to a medium bowl, stir in the flour and then tip in the squid. Toss together until the squid is well coated with the spices.

Heat the oil in a large wok over a high heat and stir-fry the squid for 2–3 minutes or until it curls up and lightly browns. Tip onto a serving platter and serve with chilli dipping sauce (see below), if you like, add a few lime wedges for squeezing over the squid.

Chilli dipping sauce: Put 25g caster sugar, 75ml of water and 1 tablespoon of white wine vinegar in a small saucepan and gently heat until the sugar dissolves, stirring continuously. Bring to the boil and cook for 1 minute. Add 1 finely chopped (and deseeded if preferred) long red chilli and 2 finely chopped garlic cloves and cook for 1 minute more, stirring occasionally. Remove from the heat and leave to cool. Serves 4. Calories per serving: 27

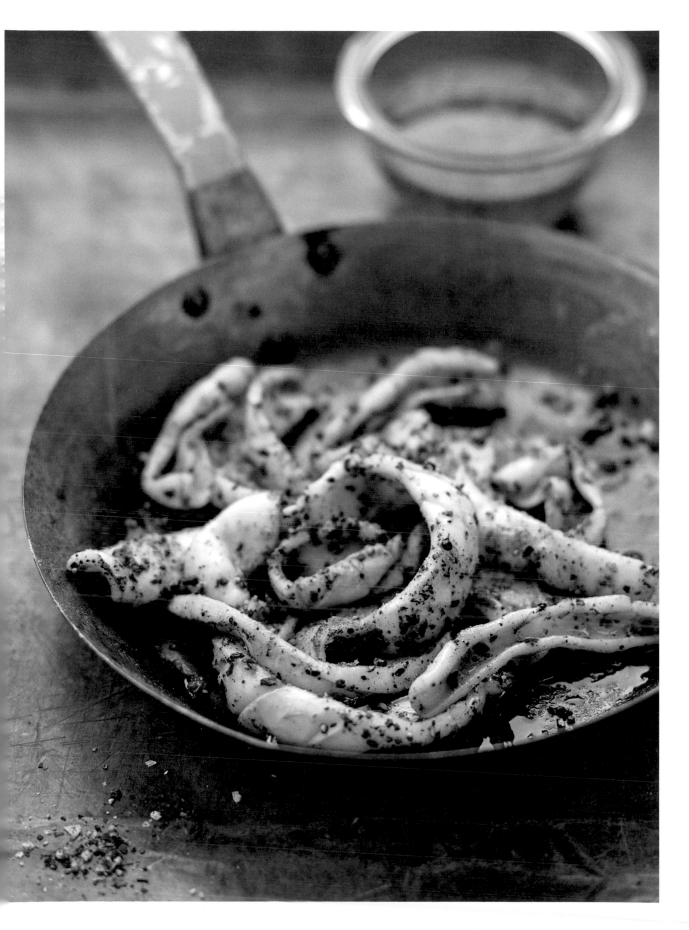

272
CALORIES
PER SERVING

king prawn stir-fry with vegetables

SERVES 2
PREP: 15 MINUTES
COOK: 5-6 MINUTES

1 tbsp sunflower oil
1 red pepper, deseeded
    and cut into 2.5cm chunks
2 large carrots, thinly sliced
125g mangetout
8 spring onions,
    cut into 2cm lengths
20g chunk fresh root
    ginger, peeled and
    very thinly sliced
2 large garlic cloves,
    very thinly sliced
1 tbsp cornflour
2 tbsp dark soy sauce
250ml chicken stock
    (made with ½ chicken
    stock cube)
200g peeled raw king
    prawns, thawed if frozen
225g can mixed bamboo
    shoots and water
    chestnuts, drained

It might seem strange to use chicken stock as a base for this dish, but it works really well, adding a savouriness that isn't at all out of place with the prawns. If you can't find any mixed cans of bamboo shoots and water chestnuts, go for plain bamboo shoots instead.

Heat the oil in a large non-stick frying pan or wok over a high heat and stir-fry the pepper and carrots for 2 minutes. Add the mangetout and cook for 1 minute more. Scatter over the spring onions, ginger and garlic and stir-fry for 1 minute.

Mix the cornflour with the soy sauce in a small bowl. Pour the chicken stock into the pan and stir in the prawns, bamboo shoots and water chestnuts and the soy sauce mixture. Bring to a simmer and cook for 1–2 minutes or until the prawns are pink throughout and glossy, stirring continuously.

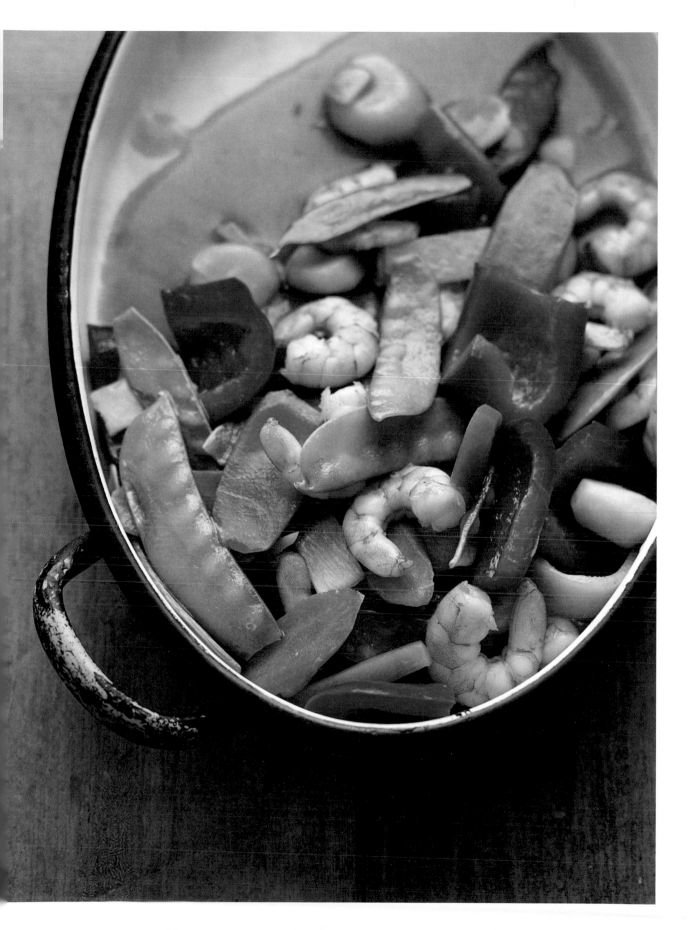

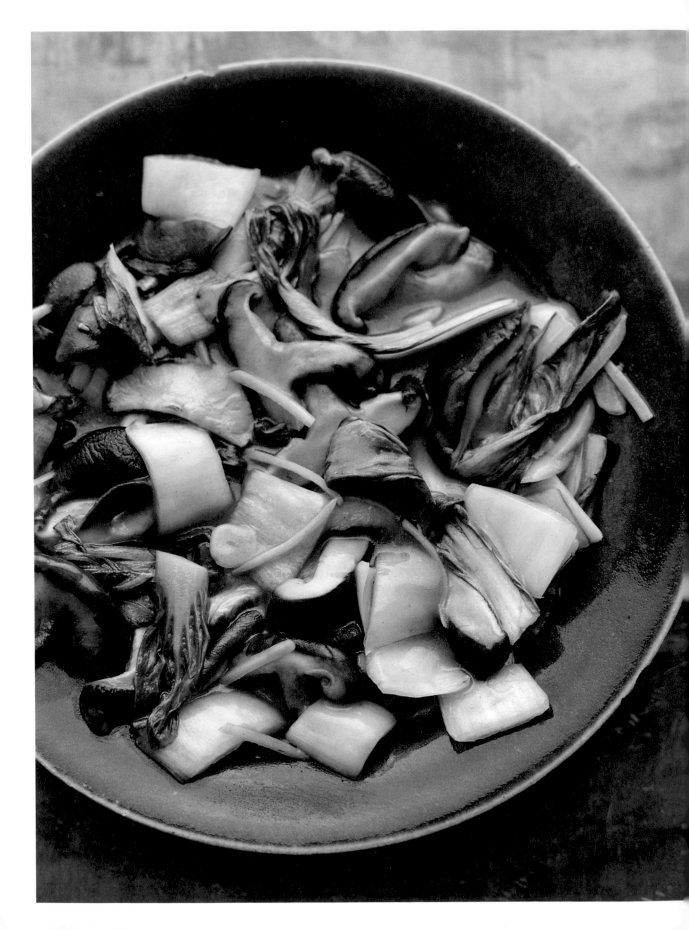

58
CALORIES
PER SERVING

stir-fried pak choi with mushrooms

SERVES 4

PREP: 15 MINUTES

COOK: 5 MINUTES

3 pak choi (about 350g), trimmed, leaves separated and washed well

1 tsp cornflour

85ml water, plus 1 tbsp

2 tbsp hoisin sauce

2 tsp sunflower oil

200g shiitake or chestnut mushrooms, wiped and thickly sliced

2 large garlic cloves, very thinly sliced

20g chunk fresh root ginger, peeled and cut into very thin matchsticks

This dish makes an ideal vegetable accompaniment and can also be used as an essential extra. Hoisin sauce is widely available and keeps in the fridge for weeks. Add a splash to any stir-fry dishes or use as a dipping sauce, but bear in mind it's high in sugar and contains around 35 calories per tablespoon, so don't go too wild.

Put the pak choi leaves on a board and cut through the white stems to separate the leafy parts. Thickly shred the stems but leave the leaves whole. Mix the cornflour with 1 tablespoon of water in a small bowl until smooth, then stir in another 85ml of water and the hoisin sauce.

Heat the oil in a large wok or non-stick frying pan over a high heat. Stir-fry the mushrooms and pak choi stems for 2 minutes, then add the garlic and ginger and cook for 1 minute more.

Drop the pak choi leaves into the pan and add the sauce. Cook over a high heat for 2 minutes, stirring regularly, or until the sauce is thickened and glossy, the pak choi leaves are wilted and the stems are just tender.

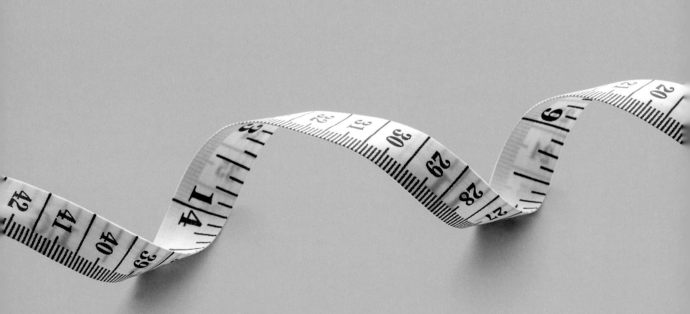

south
east asian

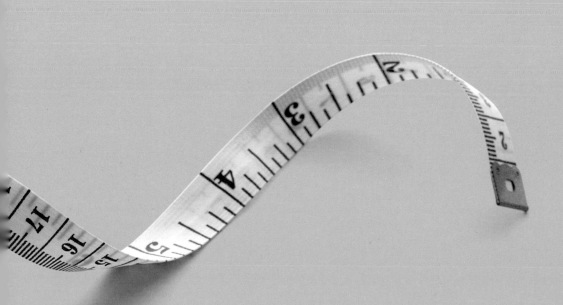

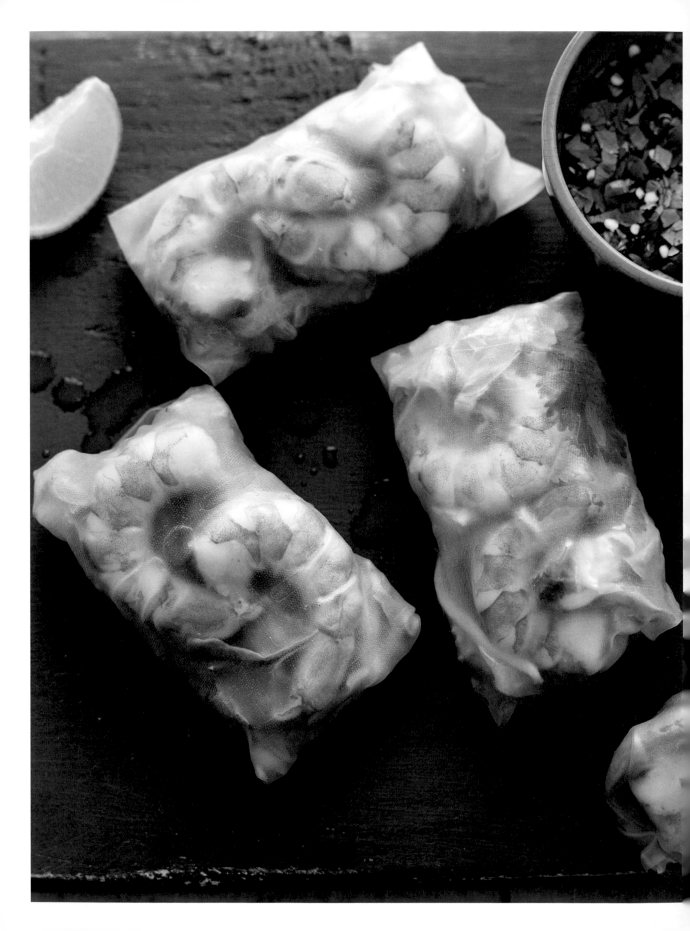

225
CALORIES
PER SERVING

vietnamese summer rolls

SERVES 4
PREP: 20 MINUTES

12 spring roll (rice pancake)
   wrappers
24 cooked and peeled
   jumbo prawns (about
   200g), thawed if frozen
   and drained
2 baby gem lettuce,
   leaves roughly shredded
6 spring onions, cut into
   very thin strips
1 medium carrot, peeled
   and coarsely grated
150g bean sprouts
10g coriander leaves,
   roughly chopped

FOR THE DIPPING SAUCE
1 tbsp Thai fish sauce
   (nam pla)
1 tbsp light soft brown sugar
2 tbsp fresh lime juice
1 red bird's eye chilli,
   thinly sliced
10g fresh coriander,
   leaves finely chopped

Summer rolls make a fresh, light meal. The rice wrappers are sold as clear hard sheets that look like plastic; when soaked in water they become soft and pliable, nearly translucent and ready to eat.

To make the dipping sauce, mix together all of the ingredients in a non-metallic bowl and set aside.

Boil a kettle full of water, then pour the water into a heatproof bowl. Leave to cool for 5 minutes. Take a spring roll wrapper and use tongs to dip it into the water for 5 seconds or until floppy. Remove it immediately and place onto a board.

Lay 2 of the prawn halves in a row in the centre of the wrapper. Place a mixture of the vegetables and a few coriander leaves on top of the prawns.

Bring the bottom end of the wrapper up over the filling and then the other end, followed by both sides. Place on a plate with the fold side down. Repeat with the remaining wrappers. Serve with the dipping sauce alongside.

265
CALORIES
PER SERVING

fragrant beef, herb and watermelon salad

SERVES 4
PREP: 20 MINUTES
COOK: 2–5 MINUTES

350g sirloin or rump steak
   (around 2cm thick),
   trimmed of hard fat
1 tsp sunflower oil
3 carrots, diagonally sliced
½ large cucumber, cut
   into 5cm-long sticks
150g radishes, halved
½ medium red onion,
   thinly sliced
½ small watermelon (about
   1.25kg), cut into wedges,
   deseeded, peeled and cut
   into 3cm chunks
40g fresh mint,
   leaves roughly torn
20g fresh coriander,
   leaves roughly torn
25g roasted, salted cashew
   nuts, broken in half
flaked sea salt
ground black pepper

FOR THE DRESSING
2 tbsp Thai fish sauce
   (nam pla)
2 tbsp, plus 1 tsp light
   soft brown sugar
2 tbsp fresh lime juice
1 or 2 red bird's eye chillies,
   trimmed and very thinly
   sliced (depending on
   how much heat you like)

This recipe is based on the classic Thai beef salad, but I wanted to make it a bit fruity and colourful, so I've added fresh watermelon. It looks fab and the combination of the chilli dressing, heaps of fragrant herbs and cooling watermelon is hard to beat.

Rub the steak all over with the oil and season with salt and lots of freshly ground pepper. Place a large non-stick frying pan over a high heat and fry for 1½–2 minutes on each side. The steak is definitely best served rare for this salad, but if your steak is quite thick, be prepared to cook it for an extra 1–2 minutes on each side. Place the steak on a board to rest while you prepare the salad.

Toss the carrots, cucumber, radishes, red onion and watermelon in a large bowl. Scatter the mint leaves, coriander and cashews over the top and turn a couple of times. Tip gently onto a serving platter.

Slice the steak into thin strips and dot around the salad. Mix together the dressing ingredients in a small bowl and drizzle over the top of the salad. Serve immediately while the steak is still warm and before the leaves have a chance to wilt.

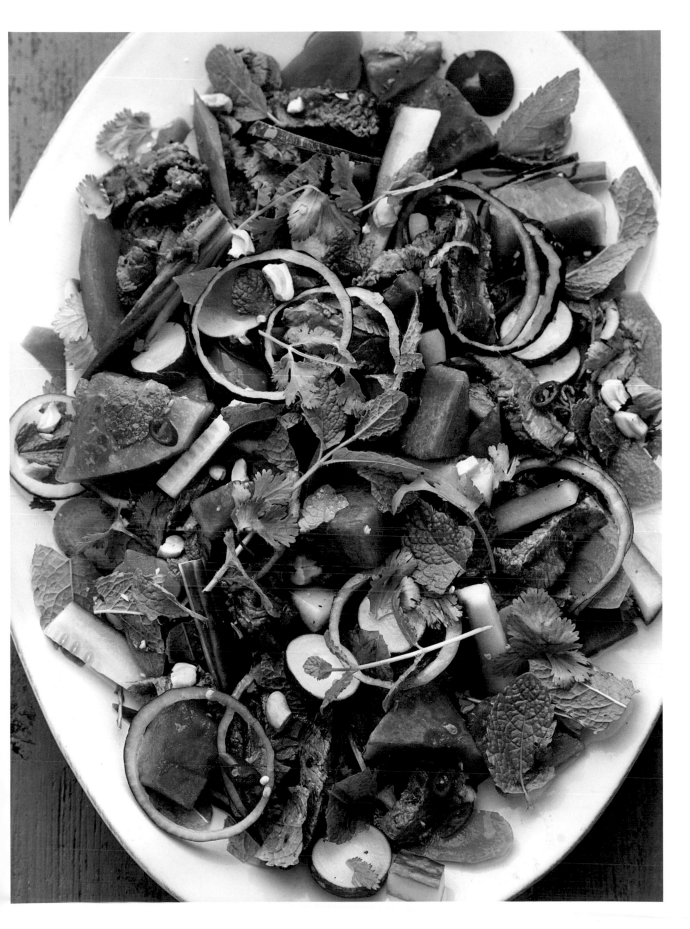

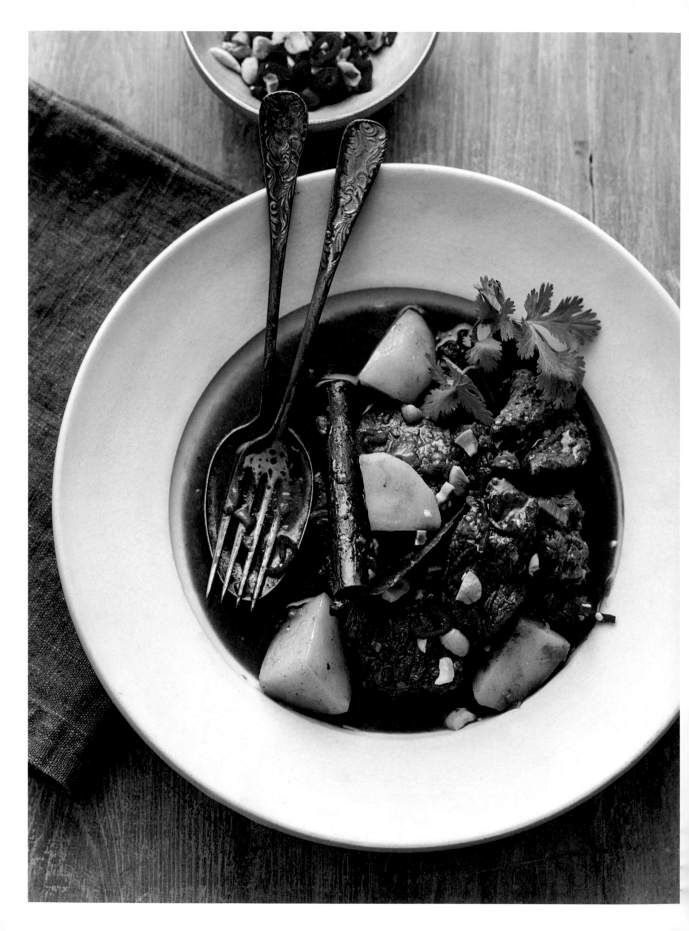

495
CALORIES
PER SERVING

beef massaman curry

SERVES 4
PREP: 15 MINUTES
COOK: 1³/₄ HOURS

800g braising beef
(ideally chuck steak)
1 tbsp sunflower oil
2 medium onions,
thinly sliced
3 tbsp good-quality
massaman curry paste
or Thai red curry paste
1 cinnamon stick
1 star anise
5 fresh, frozen or dried
Kaffir lime leaves
400ml can reduced
fat coconut milk
1 beef stock cube
2 tbsp Thai fish sauce
(nam pla)
1 tbsp light soft brown
sugar or palm sugar
2 large potatoes (about
500g), peeled and cut
into 2cm chunks
chilli peanuts (see right),
to serve (optional)

Tip: The addition of
potatoes means you don't
need to serve this dish with
rice. Add a big bowl of
green vegetables or a leafy
salad on the side instead.

Peanuts are a common feature in a massaman curry, but
by adding them as a separate sprinkle, you can keep a close
eye on the calories. Covering the surface of the curry with
baking parchment prevents moisture escaping and keeps
the beef succulent.

Preheat the oven to 170°C/Fan 150°C/Gas 3½. Trim the beef
of all hard fat and cut into roughly 2.5cm chunks. Heat the oil
in a large non-stick frying pan or wok and fry the onions over
a medium heat for 2–3 minutes until lightly browned, while
stirring. Add the beef and stir-fry together for 2 minutes
or until the beef is lightly coloured.

Stir in the curry paste, cinnamon stick, star anise and
lime leaves and cook for 1 minute, while stirring. Tip into a
flameproof casserole. Pour over the coconut milk, crumble
the beef stock cube on top and add the fish sauce and sugar.

Bring to a gentle simmer, then turn off the heat and cover
the surface of the curry with baking parchment This will
stop the curry drying out. Pop a lid on top and cook in
the oven for 45 minutes.

Take the dish out of the oven and stir in the potatoes. Cover
and return to the oven for a further 45 minutes or until the
beef and potatoes are tender. Serve sprinkled with chopped
chilli peanuts and fresh chilli if you like. (Don't eat the star
anise or the lime leaves.)

Chilli peanuts: Roughly chop 20g roasted salted peanuts
and finely slice 1 long red chilli. Mix together in a small bowl.
Sprinkle over curries, soups and salads. Serves 4.
Calories per serving: 31

146
CALORIES
PER SERVING

thai fishcakes

SERVES 4
PREP: 15 MINUTES
COOK: 20–25 MINUTES

250g skinless white fish
  fillet, such as haddock or
  cod, cut into 3cm chunks
200g raw peeled prawns,
  thawed if frozen
20g chunk of galangal
  or fresh root ginger,
  peeled and finely grated
2 garlic cloves, finely grated
4 fresh, frozen or dried
  Kaffir lime leaves,
  very thinly sliced
1 tbsp Thai fish sauce
  (nam pla)
6 spring onions, thinly sliced
1 long red chilli, deseeded
  and thinly sliced
10g fresh coriander,
  leaves finely chopped
1 tbsp sunflower oil

TO SERVE
Thai cucumber salad
  (see below)
chilli dipping sauce
  (see page 66)
lime wedges, for squeezing

Open freeze the cooked
fishcakes, pack into a
freezer-proof container
interleaving with non-stick
baking paper and return
to the freezer for up to
2 months. Reheat from
frozen in a lightly oiled
frying pan over a low
heat until piping hot.

Thai-style fishcakes make an ideal meal when you are counting
calories as they contain very little fat. I serve mine with a
pickled cucumber salad (see below), but you could also add
a green leafy salad and perhaps some new potatoes or baked
sweet potato wedges for a more substantial meal. If you can't
get hold of fresh galangal, you can opt for the ready-prepared
kind instead; you'll need 1 tablespoon of the paste.

Put the fish fillet, prawns, galangal or ginger, garlic, lime leaves
and fish sauce in a food processor and blend to a thick paste.
You may need to remove the lid and push the mixture down
a couple of times with a spatula until the right consistency
is reached.

Scrape the mixture into a bowl and stir in the spring onions,
chilli and coriander until evenly mixed. With wet hands, form
the mixture into 12 small balls and flatten into fishcakes around
1.5cm thick.

Heat the oil in a large non-stick frying pan and place over
a medium-low heat. Cook the fishcakes in 2 batches for
5–6 minutes on each side or until lightly browned and
cooked throughout. Keep the first batch warm in a low
oven while the rest are cooked.

Serve the hot fishcakes with a Thai cucumber salad, sweet
chilli dipping sauce and lime wedges for squeezing.

Thai cucumber salad: Put 1 tablespoon white wine vinegar,
1 tablespoon caster sugar and 2 teaspoons Thai fish sauce
(nam pla) in a bowl and mix with a spoon until the sugar
dissolves. Cut 1 cucumber in half lengthways and scrape out
the seeds with a teaspoon. Very thinly slice the cucumber and
add it to the dressing. Stir in 1 deseeded and finely diced long
red chilli and a handful of roughly shredded fresh mint leaves
and toss lightly together. Stand for 10 minutes before serving.
Serves 4. Calories per serving: 23

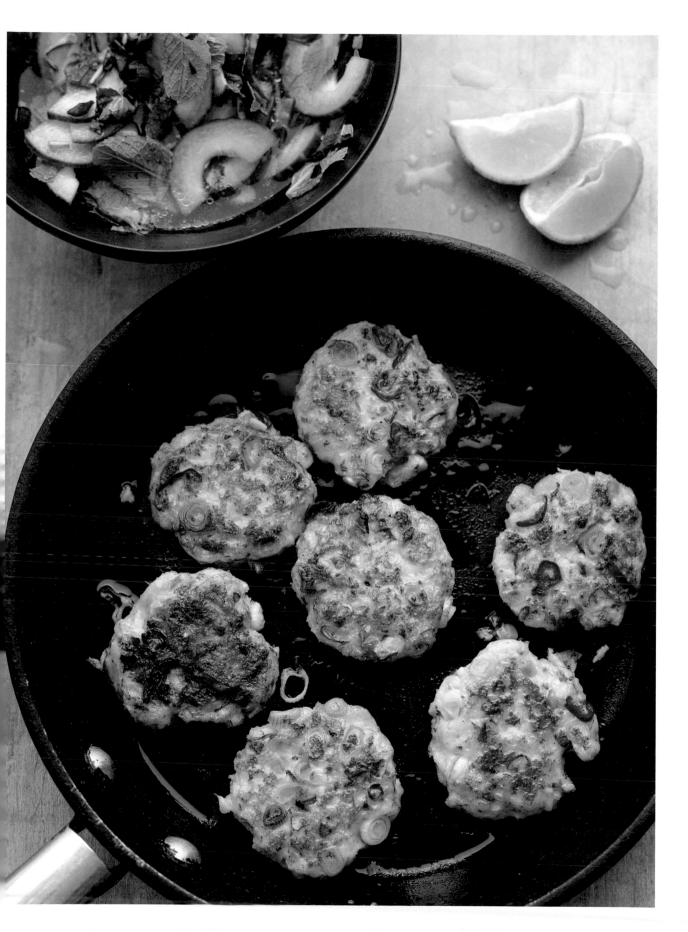

238

gado-gado chicken salad

400g baby new
   potatoes, halved
3 large fridge-cold eggs
1 head Chinese leaf, leaves
   well rinsed and cut into
   2cm-wide slices
1 small round lettuce or
   2 baby gem lettuces,
   leaves separated
1 cucumber, cut into 5cm-
   long sticks
1 large long shallot or
   5 small shallots, peeled
   and finely sliced
1 large carrot, peeled and
   coarsely grated
75g bean sprouts, rinsed
   and drained
20g fresh mint, leaves torn
   or shredded if large
400g skinless cooked
   chicken breasts (roughly
   3), torn into long strips
creamy peanut dressing
   (see right), to serve

Tips: You can always poach
your own fresh chicken
breasts if you don't want to
use the ready-cooked kind.
Simply pop the breasts into
a pan of simmering water
and cook for 12–15 minutes.

Grate the carrot into long
strips by holding it vertically
against the coarse side of
your grater – but watch
your fingers!

**This salad is my take on gado-gado, an Indonesian dish
consisting of vegetables and hard-boiled eggs, served with
a peanut sauce. I like to put the whole platter on the table
and ask people to dig in and help themselves.**

Cook the potatoes in a pan of boiling water for 15–20 minutes
or until tender. Drain, then plunge into a bowl of cold water
to cool.

Meanwhile, half fill a medium saucepan with water and bring to
the boil. Gently lower the eggs into the water and return to the
boil. Cook for 9 minutes exactly. Drain and rinse under running
water until the shells feel cold. Put the eggs in a bowl of very
cold water and set aside.

To make the salad, gently toss the Chinese leaves and
lettuce leaves (with any particularly large leaves torn in half),
cucumber, shallot, half the carrot, half the bean sprouts and
the mint leaves in a big bowl and tip gently over a large
serving platter.

Peel the eggs and cut them into quarters. Arrange the eggs
and chicken strips over the salad and scatter the rest of
the carrot and bean sprouts on top. Drizzle with a little
of the peanut dressing and serve the rest separately.

Creamy peanut dressing: Put 50g smooth peanut butter,
100ml reduced fat coconut milk, 1 tablespoon Thai sweet
chilli dipping sauce, 1 tablespoon white wine vinegar and
2 teaspoons dark soy sauce in a small saucepan and heat
gently, stirring constantly, until the sauce is smooth. Add
1–2 tablespoons cold water if the dressing seems too thick
to drizzle. Pour into a heatproof serving jug and leave to
cool. Serve over salad or use as a sauce for grilled poultry
or meat. Serves 6. Calories per serving: 67

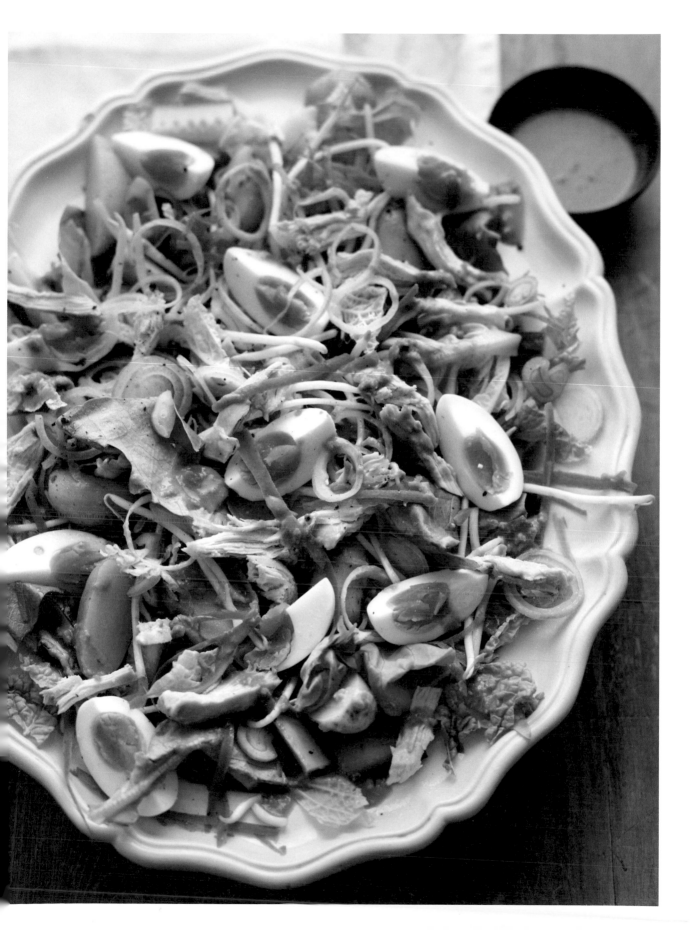

306

CALORIES
PER SERVING

thai red chicken curry

SERVES 4
PREP: 15 MINUTES
COOK: 20 MINUTES

4 boneless, skinless
  chicken breasts
3 tbsp Thai red curry paste
400ml can reduced-fat
  coconut milk
1 tbsp Thai fish sauce
  (nam pla)
6 fresh, frozen or dried
  Kaffir lime leaves
150g baby corn, trimmed
  and halved
2 red peppers, deseeded
  and cut into 3cm chunks
150g green beans, trimmed
Thai sticky rice or rice
  noodles, to serve

This is a bit milder than a typical Thai curry. You can find red curry paste in the Asian section of most large supermarkets. Red curries tend to have a deeper flavour than green curries as the pastes are made from dried red chillies instead of the fresh green chillies. Be careful not to boil the coconut milk or it may separate.

Cut the chicken breasts into roughly 2.5cm chunks. Put the curry paste in a non-stick frying pan, add the chicken and cook over a medium heat for 3 minutes, stirring until the chicken is lightly coloured on all sides.

Pour the coconut milk into the pan and stir in the fish sauce, lime leaves and all the vegetables. Bring to a gentle simmer and cook, loosely covered, for 15 minutes or until the chicken is tender.

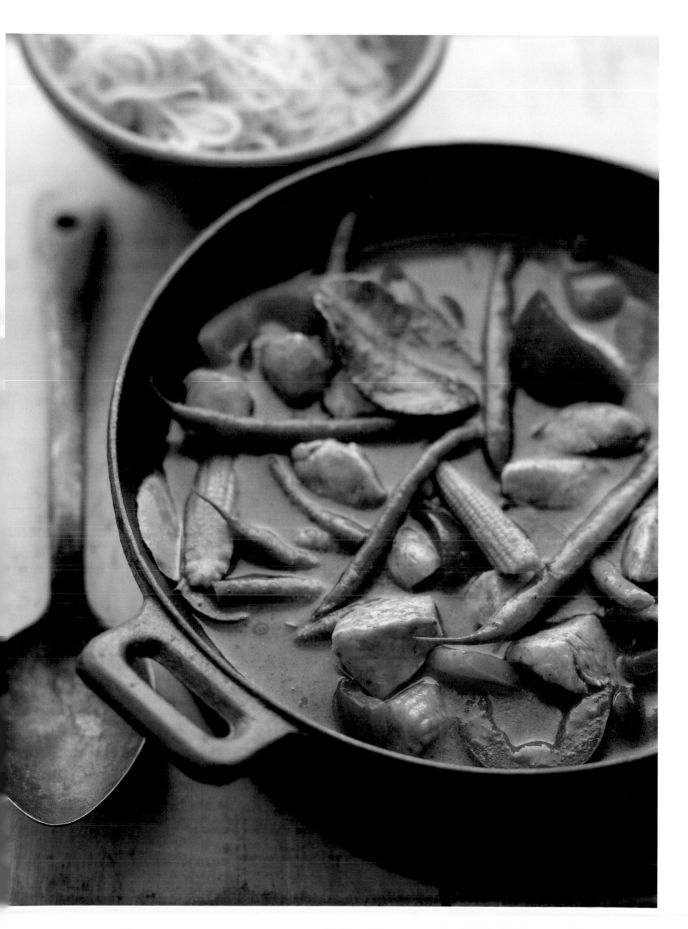

174
CALORIES
PER SERVING

simple chicken satay

SERVES 4
PREP: 30 MINUTES, PLUS MARINATING TIME
COOK: 5–8 MINUTES

3 boneless, skinless
  chicken breasts

FOR THE MARINADE
1 tbsp galangal paste
  (from a jar or tube)
1 tbsp lemongrass paste
  (from a jar or tube)
1 tbsp dark soy sauce
1 tbsp Thai fish sauce
  (nam pla)
2 tbsp fresh lime juice
1 tsp dried chilli flakes
¼ tsp ground turmeric
1 tbsp sunflower oil,
  plus extra for greasing
ground black pepper
lime wedges, for squeezing
easy satay sauce
  (see right), to serve

Open freeze the marinated chicken sticks then wrap them in tightly sealed bags and return to the freezer for up to 2 months. Cook from frozen as above, doubling the recommended time, until piping hot.

This is definitely my favourite recipe for chicken satay. The combination of succulent, lightly spiced chicken breast and tangy peanut sauce is perfect as a starter or main course served with a salad. I've used ready-made lemongrass and galangal paste for the marinade as I have been bowled over by the improvement in this type of product over the last few years.

To make the marinade, put the galangal and lemongrass paste, soy sauce, fish sauce, lime juice, chilli flakes, turmeric and oil in a bowl and season generously with black pepper. Trim the chicken of any visible fat and cut at a slight diagonal angle into long 1cm-wide strips. Add the strips to the marinade and stir well.

Thread the chicken strips onto short metal or well-soaked wooden skewers, making sure they aren't packed too tightly as the heat needs to penetrate the meat. The chicken should be fairly flat so it cooks evenly once threaded. Put the skewers on a plate, cover and marinate in the fridge for 1–4 hours.

Cook the chicken skewers on a lightly oiled and preheated griddle for 3–4 minutes on each side or until lightly charred and cooked through. Alternatively, place the skewers on a rack above a baking tray or grill pan lined with foil. Cook under a preheated hot grill for 8–10 minutes, turning once, or until lightly charred and cooked throughout.

Serve the hot satay sticks with the warm satay sauce for dipping and lime wedges for squeezing over.

Easy satay sauce: Put 2 tablespoons crunchy peanut butter in a small heatproof bowl and stir in 2 tablespoons just-boiled water until evenly mixed. Add 1 tablespoon sweet chilli sauce and stir well. Pour into a small serving bowl. Serves 4. Calories per serving: 53

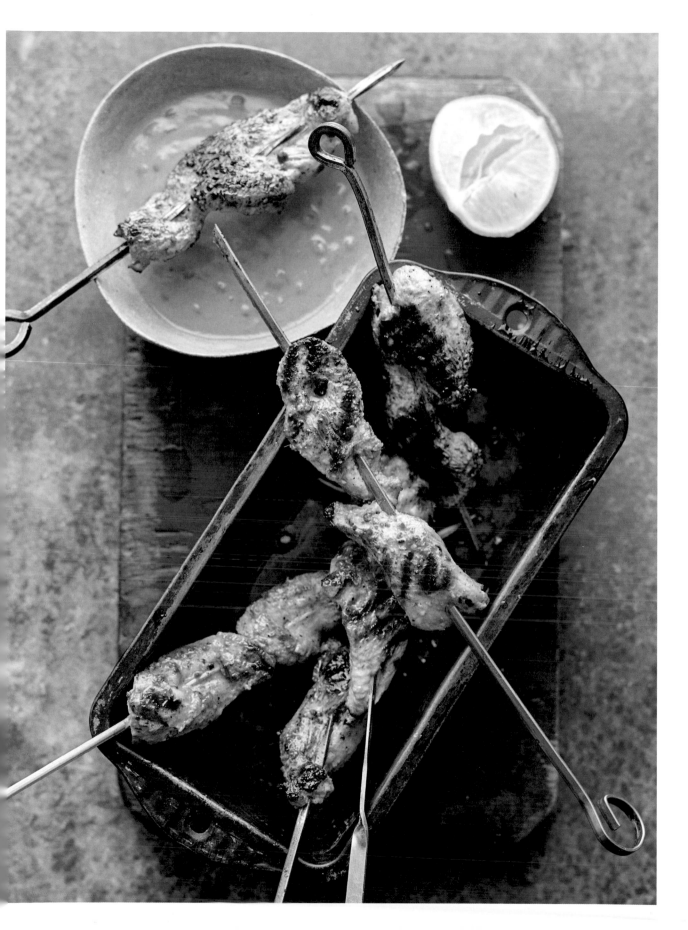

355

penang chicken and sweet potato curry

SERVES 4
PREP: 15–20 MINUTES
COOK: 30–40 MINUTES

8 boneless, skinless chicken thighs (about 650g)
3 tbsp Thai red or yellow curry paste
400ml can reduced-fat coconut milk
1 tbsp crunchy peanut butter
1 tbsp Thai fish sauce (nam pla)
4 fresh, frozen or dried Kaffir lime leaves
2 medium sweet potatoes (about 450g), peeled and cut into roughly 3cm chunks
1 tsp sunflower oil
6 shallots or 2 long banana shallots, finely sliced
fresh coriander, to garnish
stir-fried broccoli with chilli and garlic (see right), to serve

This rich and creamy curry is packed with flavour and is a doddle to make due to good-quality curry paste. The sweet potatoes add colour and are filling enough so you don't need to serve with rice. Be careful to measure the peanut butter accurately as it is very high in calories and be sure to use good-quality reduced-calorie coconut milk.

Trim the chicken of any excess fat – a pair of kitchen scissors is good for this. Cut each chicken thigh in half. Put the curry paste into a deep non-stick frying pan, add the chicken and cook over a medium heat for 4 minutes, stirring until the chicken is lightly coloured on all sides.

Pour the coconut milk into the pan, add the peanut butter, stir in the fish sauce and Kaffir lime leaves and simmer gently for 10 minutes. Add the sweet potato pieces, return to a gentle simmer, cover loosely with a lid and cook for 15–20 minutes or until the chicken is tender and the sauce is thick and glossy. Add a little extra water if necessary.

About 10 minutes before the chicken is ready, pour the sunflower oil into a small pan and fry the sliced shallots for 8 minutes, or until golden brown, stirring frequently. Serve the chicken curry topped with the fried shallots and with stir-fried broccoli.

Stir-fried broccoli with chilli and garlic: Heat 2 teaspoons sunflower oil in a large wok or non-stick frying pan and stir-fry 300g trimmed tenderstem or purple sprouting broccoli, 2 thinly sliced garlic cloves, 25g peeled and thinly sliced fresh root ginger and 1 teaspoon dried chilli flakes over a medium heat for 2 minutes. Pour over 200ml of water and steam fry the broccoli for a further 3–4 minutes until all the water has evaporated and the broccoli is just tender. Sprinkle 1 teaspoon light soft brown sugar and season with 1 tablespoon dark soy sauce and some ground black pepper. Toss together for a few seconds before serving. Serves 4. Calories per serving: 48

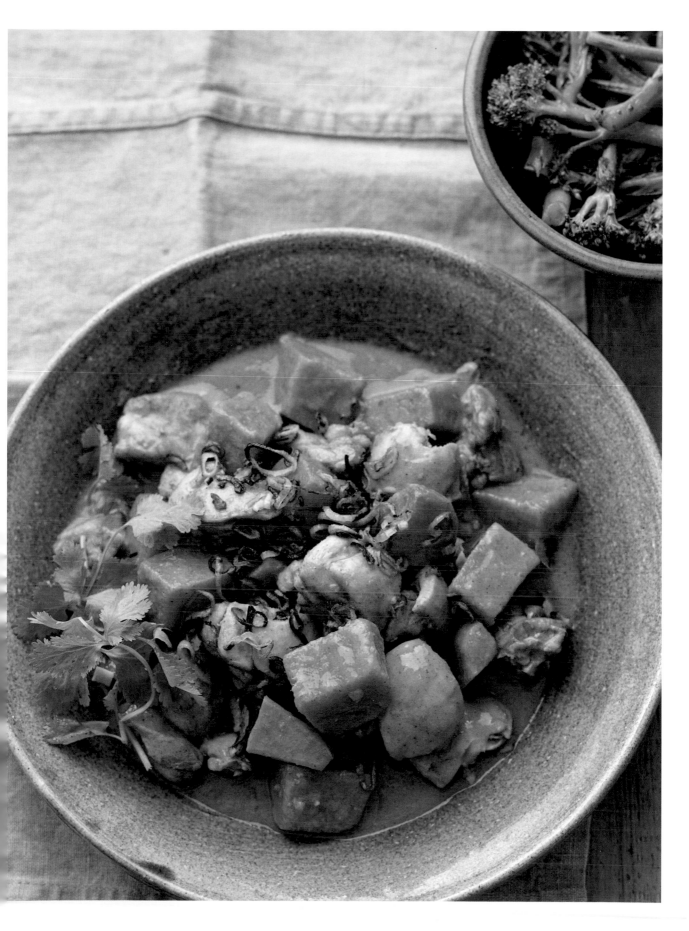

331
CALORIES
PER SERVING

jungle curry

SERVES 2
PREP: 15 MINUTES
COOK: 8-10 MINUTES

1 tsp sunflower oil
2 boneless, skinless
   chicken breasts,
   cut into small pieces
150g baby corn, trimmed
   and halved
1 red pepper, deseeded and
   cut into roughly 2cm chunks
150g mangetout
5 fresh, frozen or dried
   Kaffir lime leaves
200ml chicken stock (made
   with ½ chicken stock cube)
1 tbsp Thai fish sauce (nam pla)
large handful of fresh basil
   leaves (ideally Thai basil)
Thai sticky rice, to serve

FOR THE CURRY PASTE
2 tbsp crushed red chilli
   paste (from a jar)
20g chunk of galangal,
   peeled and chopped,
   or 1 tbsp galangal paste
   (from a jar or tube)
2 lemongrass stalks,
   chopped, or 1 tbsp
   lemongrass paste
   (from a jar or tube)
4 garlic cloves, crushed
1 tbsp sunflower oil

Freeze the cooled curry
in zip-seal bags or in foil
containers for up to
3 months. Thaw in the
fridge overnight. Reheat
in a large, wide-based
saucepan, stirring gently
until piping hot.

The chicken in this easy jungle curry needs to be cut into small pieces instead of the usual chunks or strips, so it cooks really quickly. The curry paste needs a blitz in a food processor or a good pounding with a pestle and mortar but if you use galangal and lemongrass pastes instead of the fresh variety, you can simply mix it all together in a bowl. Thai basil, sometimes known as holy basil, adds a lovely, slightly aniseed taste but you can use the common variety too. Avoid the growing basil plants that you can buy in the shop as the leaves don't contain as much flavour.

To make the curry paste, put the chilli paste, galangal, lemongrass and garlic in a food processor and add the oil. Blitz until as fine as possible. You may need to remove the lid and push the mixture down a couple of times until the right consistency is reached. If you don't have a food processor, pound everything together with a pestle and mortar.

Heat the teaspoon of oil in a large non-stick frying pan or wok and stir-fry the chicken, baby corn and red pepper for 3 minutes. Add the mangetout, Kaffir lime leaves and curry paste and fry with the chicken and vegetables for 2 minutes more.

Stir in the chicken stock and fish sauce. Bring to a simmer and cook for 2 minutes or until the vegetables are just tender. Stir in the basil leaves and serve with a small portion of Thai sticky rice. (Don't eat the lime leaves.)

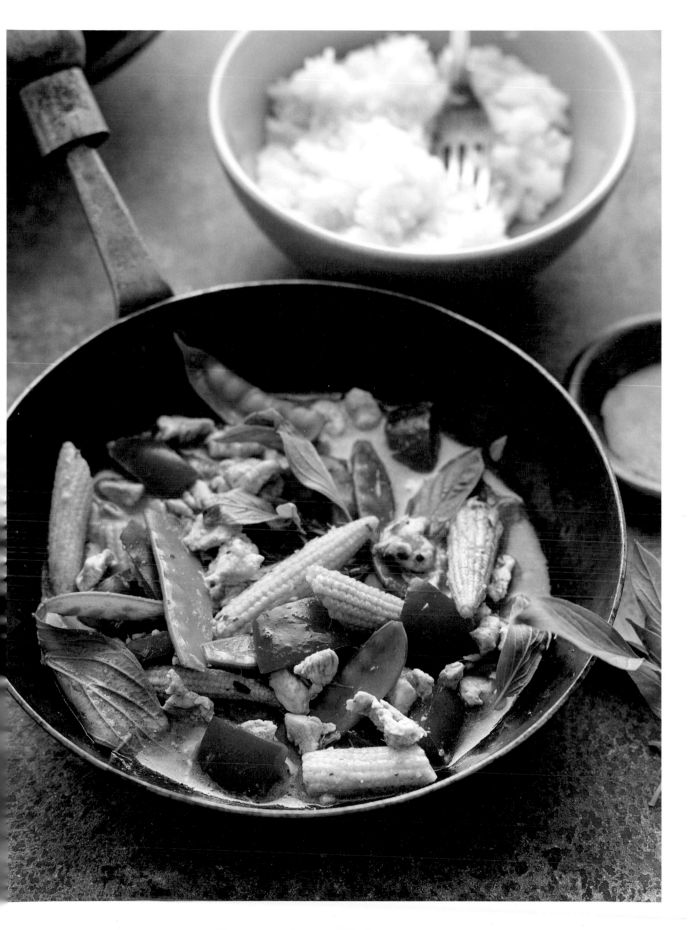

179
CALORIES
PER SERVING

prawn noodle broth

SERVES 4

PREP: 25 MINUTES

COOK: 35 MINUTES

250g raw, unpeeled king
   prawns, thawed if frozen
oil, for spraying or brushing
2 tbsp Thai red curry paste
1 medium onion, quartered
2 tbsp tomato purée
1 lemongrass stick, bruised
20g chunk fresh root ginger,
   peeled and thinly sliced
2 garlic cloves, sliced
2 bird's eye chillies, trimmed
6 fresh, frozen or dried
   Kaffir lime leaves
1 star anise
4 cardamon pods,
   lightly crushed
2 tbsp Thai fish sauce
   (nam pla)
1.5 litres cold water
100g dried flat rice noodles

This highly aromatic soup is a great light meal for a warm day that satisfyingly uses all parts of the prawns so there is no wastage. Don't be afraid to use the heads – there really is a lot of flavour in them.

Take a prawn and twist off its head. If you are lucky and pull very gently, you may be able to remove the black intestinal tract that runs down the underside of the prawn and remove it at the same time. Wipe the black tract away with a piece of kitchen paper and put the heads in a large non-stick saucepan.

Peel off the legs and shell covering the tail and place them in the pan too. If you haven't been able to remove the intestinal tract at the same time as the head, run the tip of a small knife down the side of it and flip it out. Wipe away with kitchen paper. Repeat with the rest of the prawns. Put the peeled prawns on a plate and cover with cling film. Chill in the fridge while you prepare the sauce.

Spray or brush the saucepan with oil and add the curry paste and onion to the prawn shells. Cook over a medium heat for 5 minutes, stirring and squashing the prawn shells into the base of the pan to release their flavour.

Add the tomato purée, lemongrass, ginger, garlic, chillies, Kaffir lime leaves, star anise and cardamom and cook for a few seconds, stirring. Pour over the fish sauce and the cold water and bring to a gentle simmer, stirring.

Cover loosely and simmer gently for 30 minutes, stirring occasionally. Strain the stock through a fine sieve into a clean pan – you should have about 1 litre of prawn stock for the soup.

Stir the rice noodles into the hot broth and return to a simmer. Cook for about 8 minutes or until the noodles are tender. Stir in the prawns and simmer for 1–2 minutes more or until all the prawns are fully pink, stirring every now and then. Don't overcook the prawns or they will toughen.

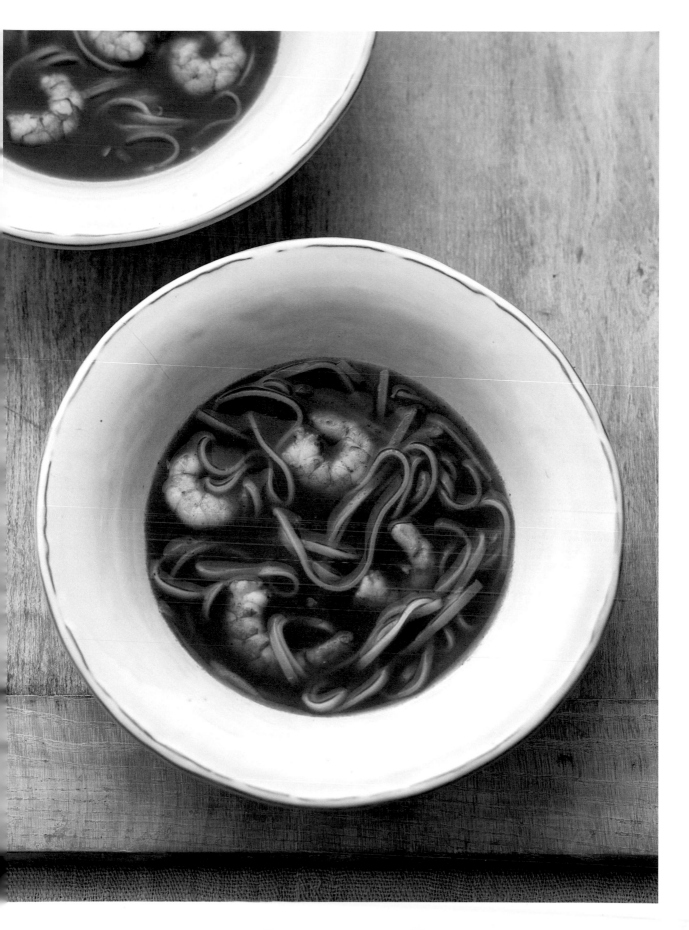

331

pad thai with prawns

SERVES 4
PREP: 20 MINUTES
COOK: 16-18 MINUTES

150g wide, flat dried
   rice noodles
1 tbsp sunflower or ground
   nut oil, plus 1 tsp
2½ tbsp Thai fish sauce
   (nam pla), plus extra
   for serving
2 tbsp fresh lime juice
1 tbsp light soft brown sugar
1 medium red onion, halved
   and cut into 12 wedges
2 garlic cloves,
   finely chopped
½ tsp dried chilli flakes
2 eggs, well beaten
175g peeled and cooked
   prawns, thawed if frozen
25g roasted salted peanuts,
   roughly chopped
8 spring onions, sliced
100g bean sprouts,
   rinsed and drained
20g fresh coriander,
   leaves roughly chopped
soy sauce, to serve

This is about as close to a takeaway pad thai as I've ever tasted. Get everything measured out and ready before you start as you need to be able to cook this dish quickly over a high heat. The slight caramelisation of the vegetables and noodles in the sweet and salty sauce is what gives the dish its deep savoury flavour.

Half fill a large saucepan with water and bring to the boil. Add the noodles in 3-4 batches and stir well after each addition. Return to the boil and cook for 3-4 minutes or until just tender. You may need to use a fork to stir the noodles as they cook.

Drain the noodles in a colander and toss with the teaspoon of oil to stop the strands sticking together, then put to one side. Mix the fish sauce, lime juice and sugar in a small bowl.

Pour the remaining tablespoon of oil into a large wok or non-stick frying pan and stir-fry the red onion over a medium heat for 2 minutes. Add the garlic and chilli flakes and cook for 30 seconds more. Push all the vegetables to one side of the pan.

Pour the beaten eggs into the pan and allow to cook into a thin omelette on the bottom. This should take 30-40 seconds. Just before the egg is completely set, use a wooden spoon to roughly chop it.

Immediately add the prawns, cooked noodles, peanuts, spring onions and fish sauce mixture. Increase the heat to its highest setting and stir-fry together for 2 minutes. Toss all the ingredients with tongs or 2 wooden spoons as you stir-fry to make sure everything is thoroughly hot and well mixed.

Add the bean sprouts and coriander and stir-fry for 2-3 minutes more or until the noodles and eggs are lightly browned in places. Divide between warmed plates or bowls using tongs. Serve with extra fish sauce and soy sauce.

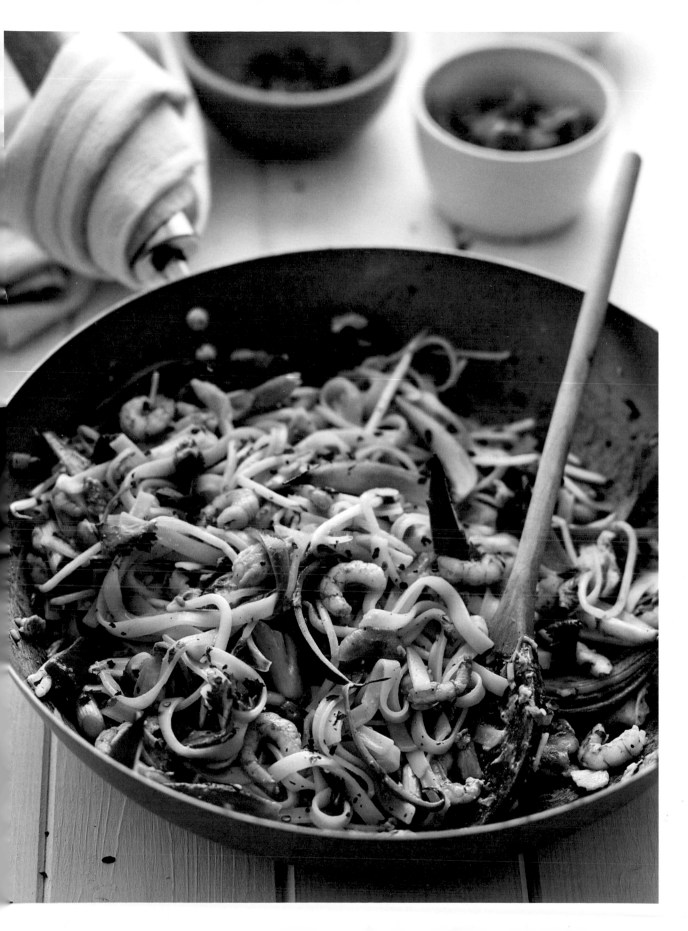

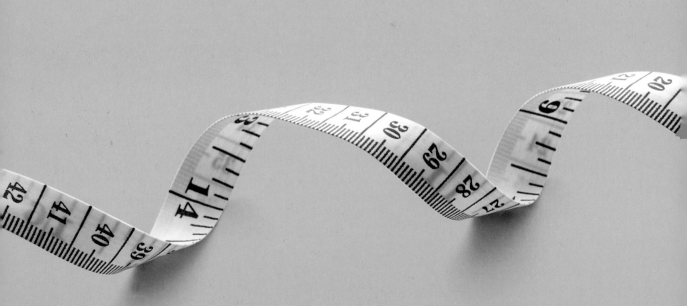

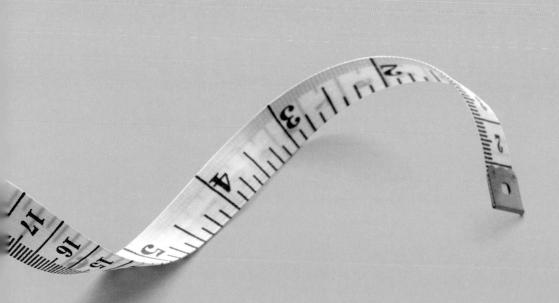

japanese

144

hand-pressed nigiri sushi

SERVES 4
PREP: 20 MINUTES,
PLUS CHILLING TIME
COOK: 30 MINUTES

700ml cold water
125g sushi rice, well
    rinsed in cold water
1½ tbsp rice vinegar
1 tsp caster sugar
1 tsp flaked sea salt
wasabi paste, to finish
12 cooked and peeled
    jumbo king prawns,
    thawed if frozen

FOR THE DIPPING SAUCE
2 tbsp dark soy sauce
2 tbsp fresh lime juice
2 tsp light soft brown sugar

TO SERVE
pickled ginger, drained
wasabi paste

Tip: Instead of prawns use
65g smoked salmon, cut
into neat rectangles. Each
piece of sushi will contain
47 calories.

Nigiri is a kind of hand-formed sushi, unlike maki, which is normally rolled using a bamboo mat. Nigiri is not covered in seaweed and is topped with only one ingredient at a time, so it is a great introduction to making sushi for complete beginners.

To prepare the rice, bring 200ml of the water to the boil in a small non-stick saucepan. Add the rice and return to the boil. Cover with a lid, reduce the heat to very low and cook for 20 minutes.

Remove the pan from the heat, keeping the lid on, and leave to stand for 10 minutes. This will allow the rice to steam and continue cooking without breaking up.

Meanwhile, mix 1 tablespoon of the vinegar, the sugar and salt together in a small bowl until the sugar has dissolved. Stir the vinegar solution into the rice until it coats every grain.

Tip the rice onto a large plate and spread out into a thin layer. Cover with cling film and leave to cool in the fridge for about 30 minutes or until completely cold.

To make the dipping sauce, mix all the ingredients together in a bowl and set aside. Run a small knife carefully down the centre of each prawn and open out.

Mix the remaining vinegar with the remaining 500ml of water in a large bowl. Dip your palms into the water. Pick up a ball of rice (around 20g) and using your hands, shape it into a small rectangle. Place it on a small board or platter. Continue with the remaining rice until you have made 12 evenly sized rectangles.

Place a dot of wasabi paste in the centre of each rectangle and drape with the prawns. Serve with the dipping sauce, pickled ginger and extra wasabi for dipping or drizzling.

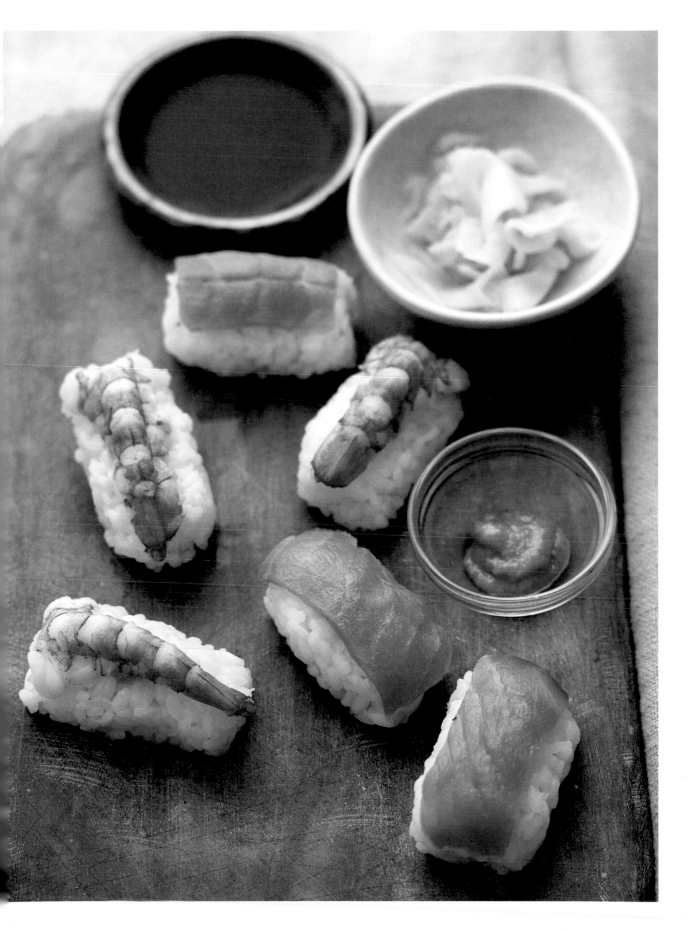

218
CALORIES
PER SERVING

maki sushi rolls

SERVES 4
PREP: 20 MINUTES,
PLUS COOLING TIME
COOK: 30 MINUTES

300ml cold water
200g sushi rice
1½ tbsp rice vinegar
1½ tsp caster sugar
1½ tsp fine sea salt
60g canned tuna in
  water, drained
1 tbsp light mayonnaise
1 tsp wasabi paste
2 sheets of sushi nori
½ small avocado, stoned,
  peeled and cut into
  5mm wide sticks
6cm length of cucumber,
  seeds removed and cut
  into 5mm wide sticks
edamame with chilli salt
  (see right), to serve

Rolling the maki may be a bit tricky to begin with, but once you've got the hang of it, it becomes almost therapeutic. This version is extra large and filled with a mixture of canned tuna, cucumber and avocado. Serve with edamame (see below), pickled ginger and dark soy sauce for dipping.

Bring the water to the boil in a small non-stick saucepan. Add the rice and return to the boil. Cover with a tight fitting lid and reduce the heat to a very low simmer. Cook for 20 minutes.

Remove the pan from the heat, keeping the lid on, and leave to stand for 10 minutes. While the rice is standing, mix the vinegar, sugar and salt in a small bowl. When the rice is ready, pour in the vinegar mixture and stir well. Tip the rice onto a large plate and spread out into a thin layer. Cover with cling film and cool in the fridge for about 30 minutes or until completely cold.

Mix the tuna, mayonnaise and wasabi paste in a bowl. Lay 1 sheet of nori on a clean board with the short end facing you. Spread half the rice over three-quarters of the nori, leaving a 5cm gap at the end furthest away from you, and smooth it out with the back of a dessert spoon. Take the spoon and press it horizontally along the middle of the rice to create a shallow groove.

Lay pieces of avocado down the groove, top with the tuna mixture and finish with cucumber sticks, all facing the same direction. Dab the uncovered nori with a little water. Take the side of the nori closest to you and start rolling away using both hands to make a fat roll. You should roll it fairly snugly, without squashing it together. Trim the ends to neaten, then cut the roll into slices. Repeat with the other sheet of nori and filling ingredients.

Edamame with chilli salt: Cook 200g of frozen edamame in boiling water for 2 minutes or until tender. Drain the beans, tip them back into a bowl and toss them with ½ teaspoon of flaked sea salt and ½ teaspoon dried chilli flakes. To eat, pop the beans out of the pods and into your mouth, discarding the pods. Serves 2. Calories per serving: 134

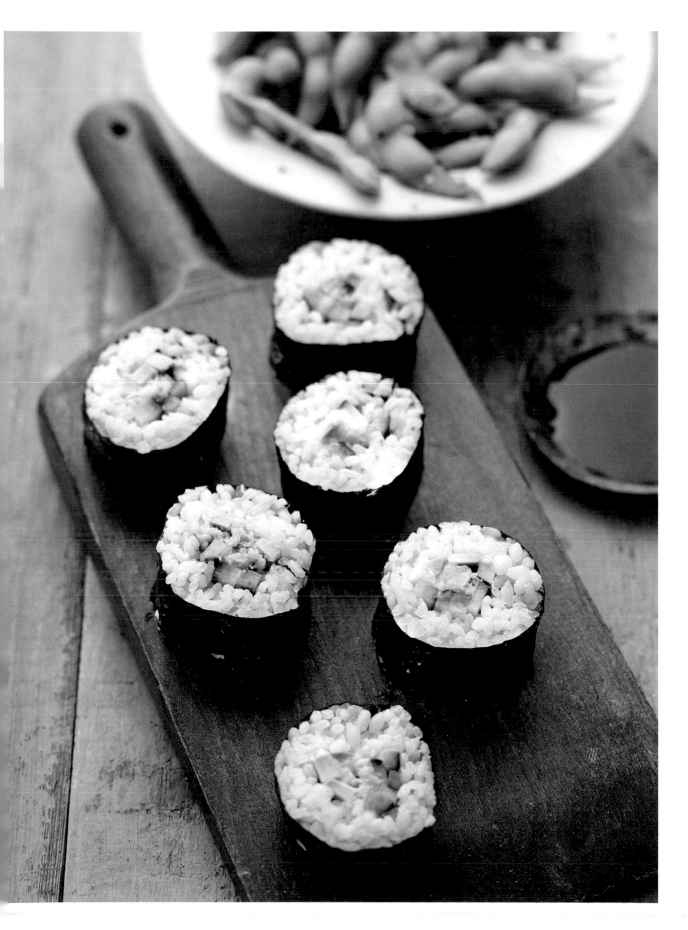

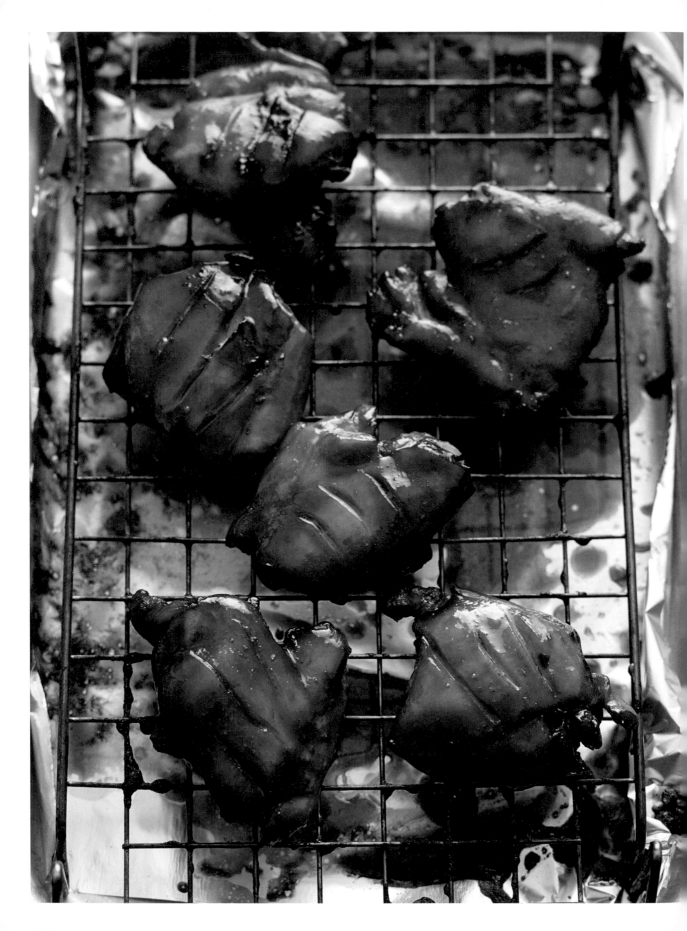

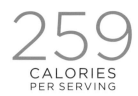

teriyaki chicken

SERVES 4
**PREP: 5–10 MINUTES,
PLUS MARINATING TIME**
COOK: 18–20 MINUTES

8 boneless, skinless chicken
thighs (about 650g)

FOR THE MARINADE
2 tbsp dark soy sauce
2 tbsp dark soft brown
sugar
2 tbsp mirin (rice wine)
or dry sherry

FOR THE BASTING SAUCE
2 tbsp clear honey
2 tbsp dark soy sauce
3 tbsp mirin (rice wine)
or dry sherry

Freeze the uncooked
marinated chicken pieces
in a zip-seal bag for up to
2 months. Thaw overnight
in the fridge and cook
according to the recipe.

Teriyaki is a simple method of cooking marinated meats while basting with a soy-based sauce. This chicken has a rich, glossy colour and deep savoury flavour. It can be served warm or cold with a small portion of rice or a large salad. Leftover chicken can be sliced and piled into lettuce wraps or tossed through a stir-fry.

To make the marinade, put the soy sauce, sugar and mirin or sherry in a large bowl and stir until the sugar dissolves. Trim the chicken thighs of any visible fat and slash each thigh 2–3 times through the thickest part with a knife. Add the chicken to the marinade, stir well, then cover and leave to marinate in the fridge for 1–4 hours.

To make the basting sauce, put the honey, soy sauce and mirin or sherry in a small saucepan and bring to the boil. Cook for 2–3 minutes, or until the sauce is thick enough to lightly coat the back of the spoon, stirring occasionally. It will continue to thicken as it cools. Remove from the heat and set aside to cool completely.

Preheat the grill to high. Drain the chicken in a sieve and arrange the pieces on a rack above a grill pan lined with foil. Tuck the chicken into neat shapes and brush generously with one-third of the basting sauce. Cook under the hot grill for 4 minutes.

Turn the chicken over and brush with half the remaining basting sauce. Return to the grill and cook for a further 4 minutes, then turn and baste again. Cook the chicken for a final 3–5 minutes or until it is cooked through and the sauce is glossy and slightly blackened in places.

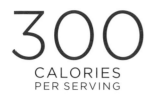

chicken katsu curry

SERVES 4
PREP: 20 MINUTES
COOK: 50 MINUTES

4 boneless, skinless chicken breasts (each about 175g)
50g panko breadcrumbs or dry coarse white breadcrumbs
½ tsp paprika (not smoked)
¼ tsp ground turmeric
4 tbsp fat-free natural yoghurt
flaked sea salt
ground black pepper

FOR THE SAUCE
oil, for brushing or spraying
2 medium onions, finely chopped
4 garlic cloves, finely chopped
20g chunk fresh root ginger, peeled and finely chopped
1 tbsp medium curry powder
½ tsp ground star anise
¼ tsp ground turmeric
400ml chicken stock (made with 1 chicken stock cube)
2 tsp tomato purée
1 tsp caster sugar

Open freeze the coated, uncooked chicken and pack into a freezer-proof container, interleaving with baking parchment. Freeze for up to 3 months. Cook from frozen as instructed, increasing the cooking time by 12–15 minutes or until the chicken is piping hot. Freeze the sauce for 3 months. Reheat gently in a saucepan from frozen until piping hot.

Chicken katsu curry is one of those dishes that everyone seems to love – especially kids. My katsu isn't fried but coated in breadcrumbs on one side, spritzed with low-calorie cooking spray and baked in the oven until crisp and golden.

To make the sauce, spray or brush a medium non-stick saucepan with oil and add the onions, garlic and ginger. Cover the pan and fry gently for 10 minutes or until well softened, stirring occasionally. Remove the lid, increase the heat a little and cook for 2–3 minutes more, or until the onions are pale, golden brown.

Stir the curry powder, ground star anise, turmeric and a good grind of black pepper into the onions. Cook for 2 minutes more, while stirring. Add the chicken stock, tomato purée and sugar, stirring continuously.

Bring the sauce to a simmer and cook for 10 minutes, stirring occasionally. Remove the pan from the heat and blitz the sauce with a stick blender until very smooth (or leave to cool for a few minutes, then purée in a food processor).

Preheat the oven to 220°C/Fan 200°C/Gas 7. Place the chicken breasts, one at a time, on a board and cover with a sheet of cling film. Bash each breast with a rolling pin until it is around 2cm thick all over. Place the chicken on a baking tray lined with baking parchment. Mix the breadcrumbs with the paprika, turmeric, a good pinch of salt and lots of black pepper.

Brush the yoghurt thickly over the top of each chicken breast and sprinkle neatly with the crumbs, pressing the crumbs into the yoghurt. Spray the chicken breasts with oil and bake them in the oven for 20 minutes or until nicely browned and cooked through, spraying with a little more oil halfway through.

About 5 minutes before the chicken is ready, bring the curry sauce to a gentle simmer and cook for 2 minutes, stirring constantly. Season to taste. Slice the crisp chicken breasts thickly and serve with the warm sauce.

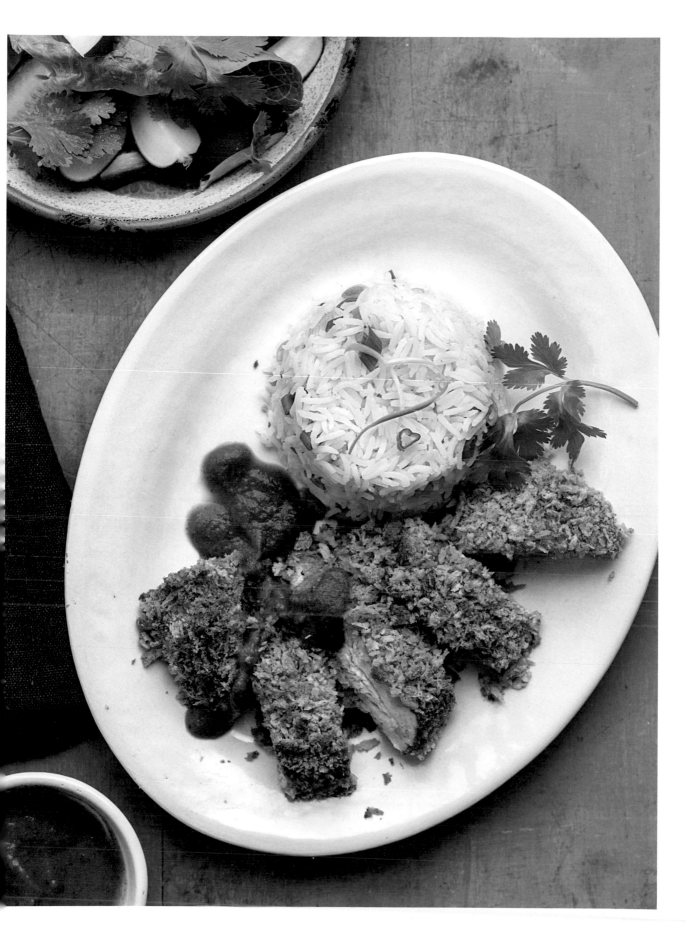

475
CALORIES
PER SERVING

ginger chicken
with udon noodles

SERVES 2

**PREP: 15 MINUTES,
PLUS MARINATING TIME**

COOK: 6–8 MINUTES

4 boneless, skinless chicken
thighs (about 325g)
1 tbsp dark soy sauce
1 tbsp freshly squeezed
lemon juice
1 tsp Chinese five-spice
powder
2 x 150g ready-to-stir-fry
cooked udon noodles
1 tsp sunflower oil
6 spring onions, cut
into 2cm lengths
2 garlic cloves,
very thinly sliced
1½ long red chillies,
very thinly sliced
½ tsp dried chilli flakes
1 egg, beaten
25g pickled ginger, drained
15g fresh coriander, leaves
roughly chopped, plus
extra to garnish
flaked sea salt
ground black pepper

This combination of fat udon noodles with gently spiced
chicken, red chilli and pickled ginger is something that I used
to drive miles to eat. I've now been able to recreate it at home
and it not only tastes better but I've also cut the calories by
a massive 200 per serving.

Trim the chicken of all visible fat and cut it into 1.5cm wide
strips. Put the chicken in a large bowl and add the soy sauce,
lemon juice and five-spice powder. Stir well and leave to
marinate for 15 minutes. Meanwhile, put the noodles in a
heatproof bowl and cover with just-boiled water from the
kettle. Leave to stand for 10 minutes, stirring to separate
the strands. Drain well in a colander.

Heat the oil in a large wok or non-stick frying pan over a
high heat and stir-fry the chicken for 1 minute or until lightly
coloured all over. Add the drained noodles, spring onions,
garlic, fresh and dried chillies to the pan and stir-fry for a
further 2 minutes.

Push the chicken and noodles to the side of the wok. Add
the egg and cook for 30–40 seconds or until almost set,
before breaking it into strands and tossing it through the
other ingredients.

Scatter the pickled ginger and chopped coriander over the
top and continue to stir-fry for 2–3 minutes more. The noodles
will be lightly browned in places and the whole dish should
smell slightly toasted when it is done. Pile into shallow bowls
and garnish with a few more sprigs of coriander.

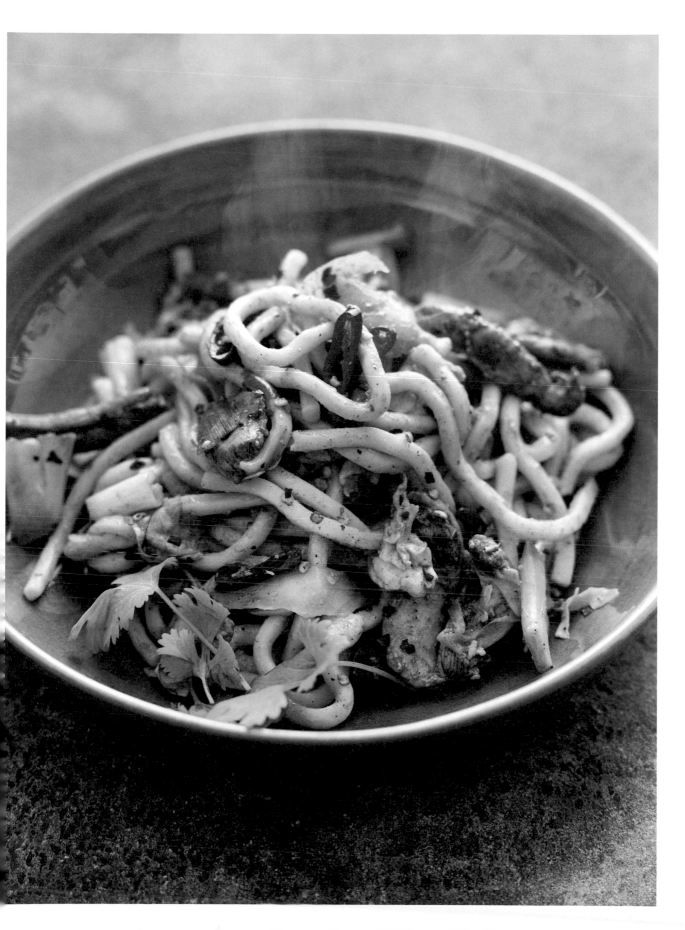

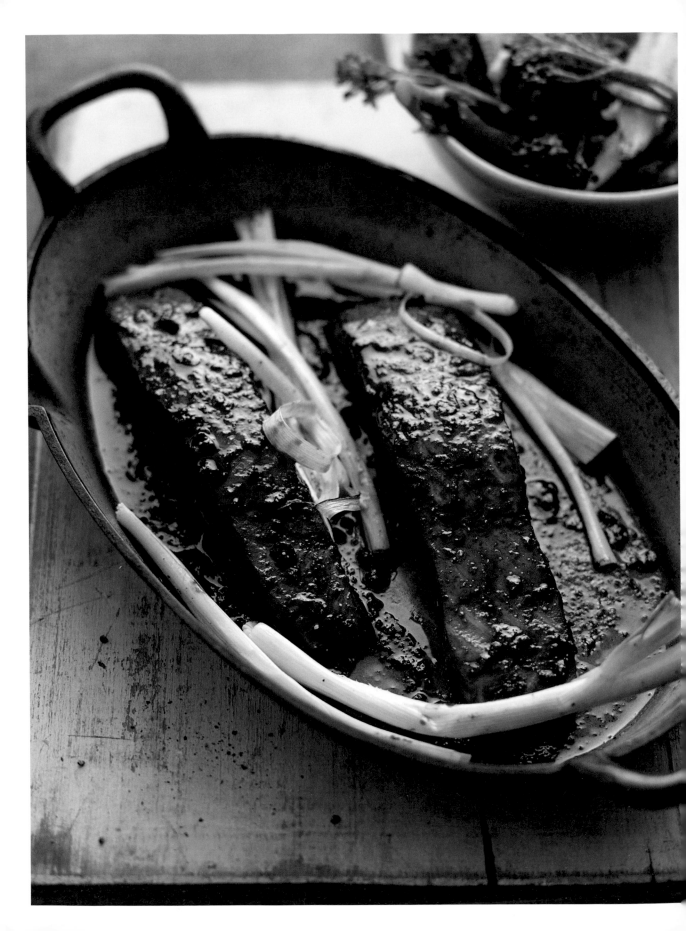

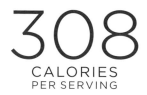
sticky miso salmon

SERVES 4

**PREP: 5 MINUTES,
PLUS MARINATING TIME**

COOK: 12-14 MINUTES

1 tbsp dark soy sauce
1 tbsp mirin (rice wine)
   or dry sherry
2 tbsp brown miso paste
1 tbsp clear honey
4 thick skinless salmon
   fillets (each about 150g)
1 tsp sunflower oil,
   for greasing
4 spring onions,
   halved lengthways

Freeze the marinated
but uncooked salmon
fillets in a zip-seal bag
for up to 2 months. Thaw
in the fridge overnight
and cook according to
the recipe.

Tip: A spoonful of miso
paste stirred into hot
chicken or vegetable
stock with some shredded
vegetables and noodles
makes a quick and
satisfying low-calorie soup.

Miso paste is a Japanese seasoning made by fermenting soya beans. It might sound a bit strange if you've never tried it, but it's an ingredient that brings the most amazing, intense flavour to this simple baked salmon and it's something I always have in my fridge. You'll find miso in the Japanese section of most large supermarkets.

Mix the soy sauce, mirin or sherry, miso and honey together in a large bowl. Add the salmon and turn in the marinade 2–3 times until the salmon is completely coated. Leave to marinate in the fridge for 30–60 minutes.

Preheat the oven to 200°C/Fan 180°C/Gas 6. Lift the salmon fillets out of the marinade, shaking off any excess, and place them in a lightly oiled, shallow ovenproof dish. Reserve the rest of the marinade. Arrange the spring onions around the salmon and bake for 8 minutes.

Take the salmon out of the oven and brush generously with the reserved marinade. Return to the oven for a further 4–6 minutes or until the salmon is just cooked and the sauce is glossy and deeply browned in places.

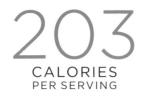

203
CALORIES
PER SERVING

pork and ponzu dressing

SERVES 4
PREP: 10 MINUTES,
PLUS MARINATING TIME
COOK: 22–25 MINUTES

500g pork tenderloin (fillet)
3 tbsp dark soy sauce or
   tamari soy sauce
2 garlic cloves, thinly sliced
oil, for brushing or spraying

PONZU DRESSING
100ml mirin (rice wine)
   or dry sherry
75ml dark soy sauce
1 tbsp rice vinegar
1 x 13cm strip of kombu
   (dried seaweed)
2 tbsp fresh lemon juice,
   plus 1–2 tsp extra, to taste
¼ tsp sesame seeds

Ponzu is a tangy Japanese sauce made from citrus and soy. Traditionally served with grilled meats, the dressing also perks up the mild flavour of pork. Serve with stir-fried vegetables and rice.

Trim as much excess fat and sinew from the pork fillet as possible, then cut in half widthways. Put the pork in a bowl and toss with the soy sauce and garlic. Cover and leave to marinate in the fridge for 1 hour.

To make the ponzu dressing, put the mirin or sherry, soy sauce, vinegar and kombu into a saucepan and bring to a simmer. Cook for 3 minutes or until reduced by almost half, stirring occasionally.

Remove the pan from the heat and leave to cool. When the liquid has cooled, remove the kombu and stir in the lemon juice and sesame seeds. (Add a little extra lemon juice if necessary just before serving – you want the dressing to taste very zingy.) Pour into dipping bowls to be served with the pork.

Preheat the oven to 200°C/Fan 180°C/Gas 6. Drain the pork well in a colander, reserving the marinade. Brush or spray a small baking tray with oil. Add the pork and bake for 18–20 minutes or until lightly browned and cooked through, brushing with the reserved marinade halfway through cooking.

Rest the pork for 10 minutes on the tray, then transfer to a board and slice. Serve with the ponzu sauce for dipping or drizzling.

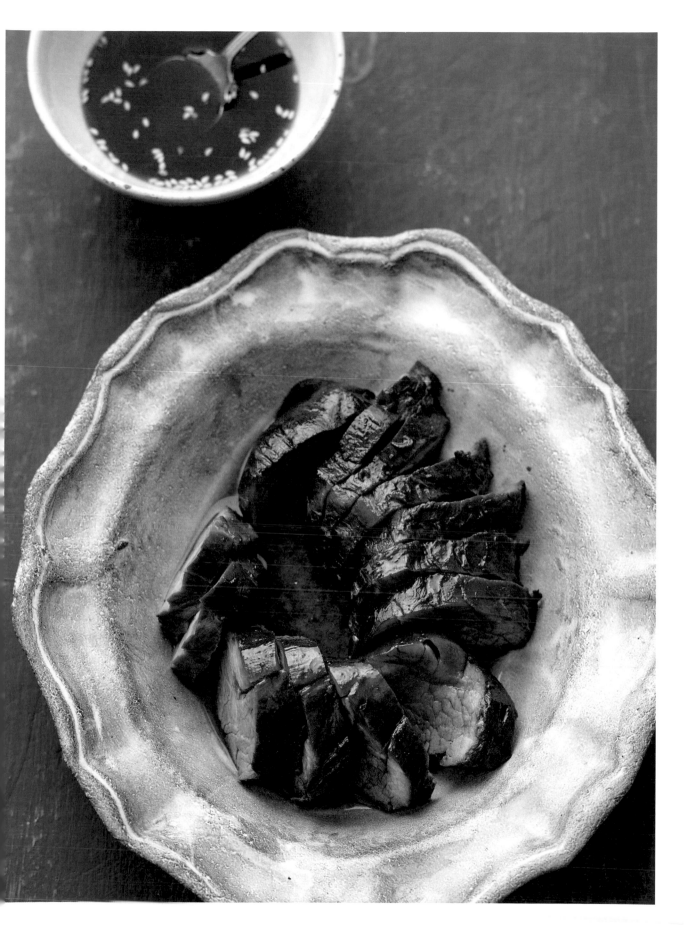

172
CALORIES
PER SERVING

ginger miso aubergines

SERVES 2
PREP: 5-10 MINUTES
COOK: 27 MINUTES

2 aubergines
oil, for spraying or brushing
50g brown miso paste
25g chunk fresh root ginger,
    peeled and finely grated
1 tbsp light soft brown sugar
4 tbsp mirin (rice wine)
    or dry sherry
4 tsp dark soy sauce
½ tsp sesame seeds

It can be difficult to get the silky texture from aubergines without plenty of oil but I think I've managed to achieve that with this recipe. Rich in savoury umami flavour from the miso and soy, the aubergines are delicious served with colourful stir-fried vegetables or my Thai cucumber salad (see page 80).

Preheat the grill to its hottest setting. Halve the aubergines and cut a criss-cross pattern into the flesh without cutting through the skin. Spray or brush a baking tray with oil and place the aubergines cut-side down. Cook under a medium-hot grill for 7–10 minutes on each side or until well softened but not burnt.

Meanwhile, mix the miso, ginger, sugar, mirin or sherry and soy sauce in a small saucepan. Bring to a gentle simmer and cook for 2 minutes, stirring regularly.

Brush the miso mixture over the cut side of the aubergines, sprinkle with sesame seeds and return to the grill for 1–2 minutes or until bubbling. Cool slightly before eating as the miso will be sticky and very hot. Serve warm.

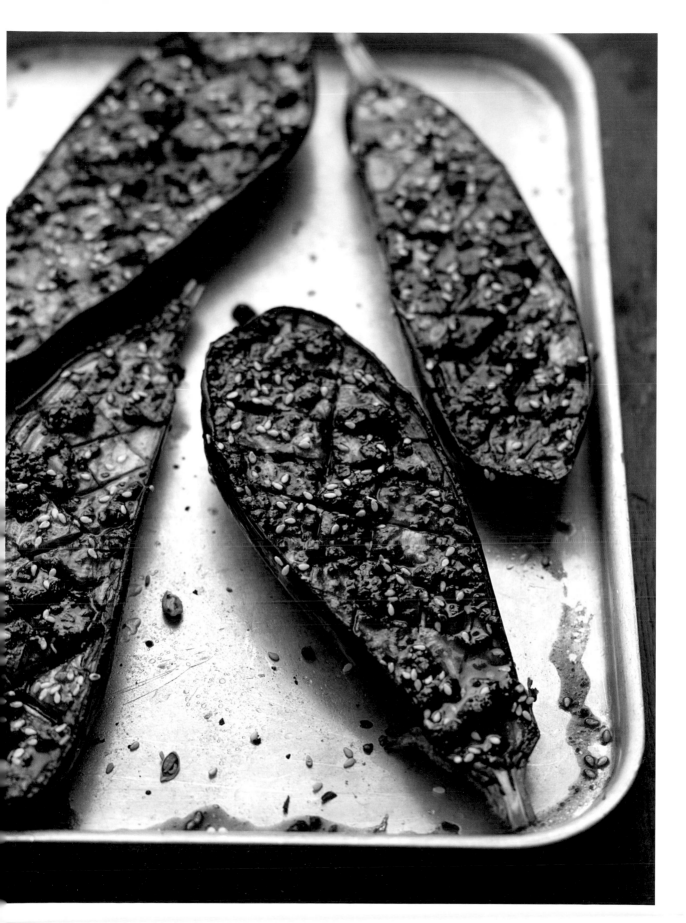

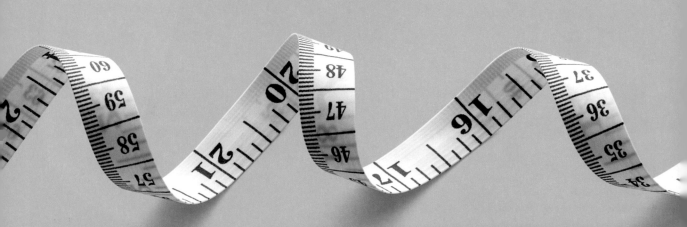

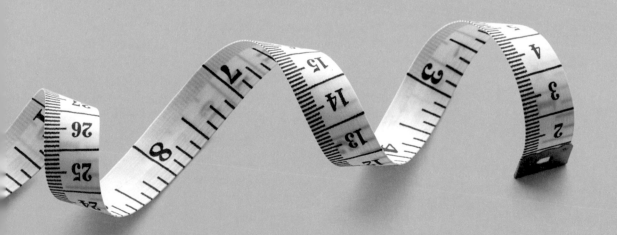

mediterranean

133
CALORIES
PER SERVING

red pepper hummus and pitta crisps

SERVES 6
PREP: 8-10 MINUTES

1 tsp olive oil
1 red pepper, deseeded
   and sliced into thin strips
1 garlic clove
large pinch dried chilli flakes
400g can chickpeas,
   drained and rinsed
1 tbsp freshly squeezed
   lemon juice
flaked sea salt
freshly ground black pepper

FOR THE PITTA CRISPS
2 large pitta breads
   (each about 85g)
oil, for brushing or spraying
1 bushy thyme sprig,
   leaves removed
1 rosemary stalk,
   leaves removed

Mezze is a popular way of eating in the Mediterranean, with lots of little plates and dips. Serve the dips with pitta crisps and lots of crunchy vegetables.

Heat the oil in a small saucepan over a medium-high heat. Add the pepper, cover with a lid and fry for 10 minutes. Remove the lid every few minutes and stir, adding a splash of water if it is beginning to stick. Add the garlic and chilli flakes. Cook for another 2–3 minutes or until the pepper is soft.

Remove the pan from the heat, add half the chickpeas to the pan and blitz with a stick blender until almost smooth. Add the remaining chickpeas, lemon juice and lots of salt and pepper. Blend until almost smooth. Cool then adjust the seasoning.

To make the pitta crisps, cut the pitta bread into stips and place on a baking tray. Spray with a little oil and season with salt and pepper. Finely chop the herbs and scatter on top. Bake in a preheated oven at 220°C/Fan 200°C/Gas 7 for 10 minutes or until crisp and golden.

Baba ganoush: Preheat the oven to 220°C/Fan 200°C/Gas 7. Halve 2 aubergines and make a few incisions into the flesh side with a sharp knife. Cut 3 garlic cloves into 4 slices each and push them deep into the flesh. Brush very lightly with oil and bake, flesh side up, on a baking tray for 35 minutes or until golden brown and very soft. When cool enough to handle, scoop the flesh into a food processor and add 1 tablespoon tahini and 2 tablespoons fresh lemon juice. Blitz until almost smooth. Serve when cool, sprinkled with a few lightly toasted cumin seeds. Serves 6. Calories per serving: 30

Minted beetroot dip: Blitz 300g drained and quartered cooked beetroots, 3 tablespoons fat-free natural yoghurt, 1 tablespoon mint sauce, 1 tablespoon extra virgin olive oil, ½ teaspoon ground cumin, and ½ teaspoon flaked sea salt and plenty of ground black pepper in a food processor until smooth. Chill before serving. Serves 6. Calories per serving: 46

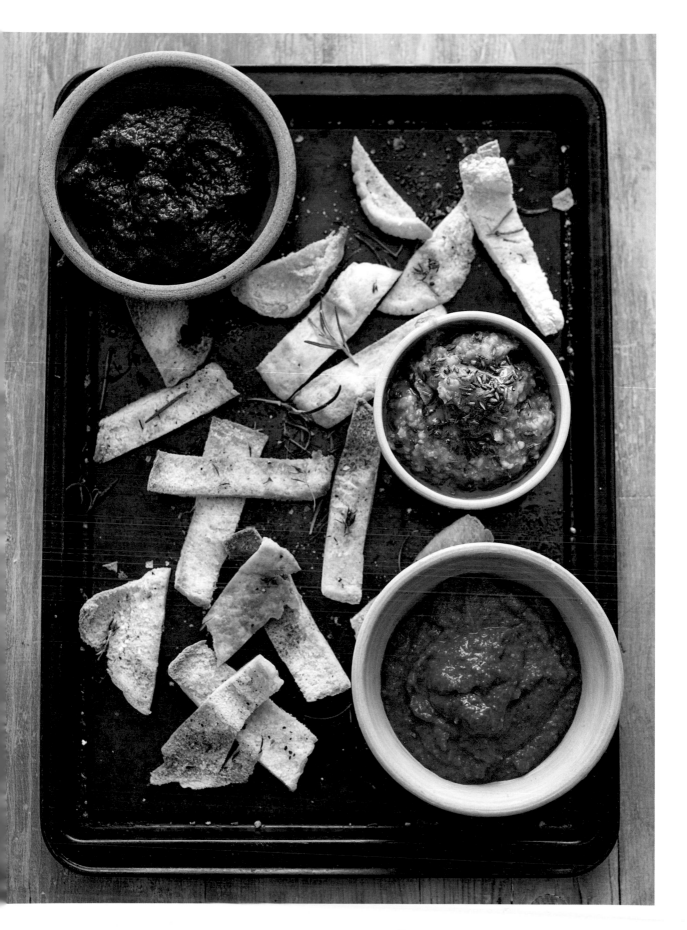

63
CALORIES
PER SERVING

moroccan marinated olives

SERVES 4

PREP: 5-10 MINUTES, PLUS MARINATING TIME

1 tbsp harissa (ideally rose harissa)
1 garlic clove, crushed
1 tsp extra virgin olive oil
2 strips orange zest
2 tbsp fresh orange juice
150g drained pitted green or black olives (in brine)

Flat freeze the marinated olives in zip-seal bags, after removing as much air as possible. To serve, tip the olives out of the bag and thaw at room temperature for 1–2 hours.

A good way of pepping up plain olives, but make sure you buy brined olives, not olives in oil. They are delicious served with my low fat tortilla chips (below). Serving everything here would bring around 270 calories per person to the table. You could also serve individual dishes as snacks for your essential extras allowance.

To make the harissa olives, mix the harissa with the garlic and olive oil and stir in the orange zest and juice and the olives. Leave to marinate in the fridge for at least 1 hour before serving.

Pesto olives: Mix 150g drained pitted green or black olives (in brine) with 2 tablespoons fresh basil pesto in a small bowl. Chill in the fridge for 1 hour before serving. Serves 4. Calories per serving: 71

Marinated feta and sun-blush tomatoes: Put ½ finely sliced red onion and 1 tablespoon white wine vinegar in a bowl and leave to stand for 30 minutes. Cut 75g feta cheese into small cubes. Drain the onion and toss very lightly with the feta, 100g drained sun-blush tomatoes and 1 tablespoon fresh thyme leaves. Serves 4. Calories per serving: 92

Low fat tortilla chips: Cut 1 large tortilla (about 60g) into small triangles using kitchen scissors and place on a baking tray. Spray lightly with oil and bake in a preheated oven at 200°C/Fan 180°C/Gas 6 for 10 minutes or until crisp and lightly golden. Serves 4. Calories per serving: 43

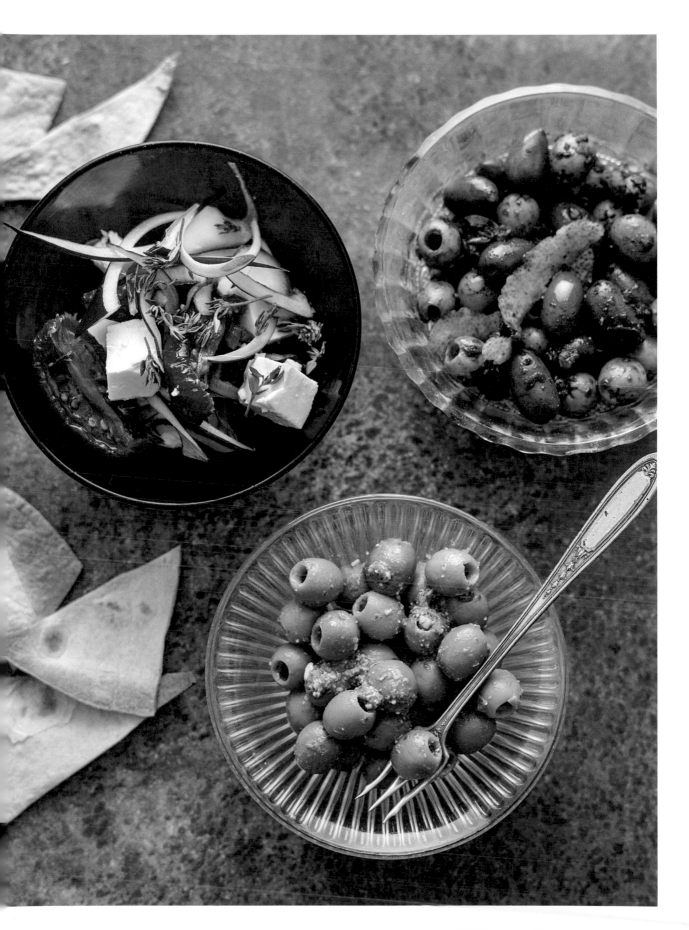

163
CALORIES
PER SERVING

bruschetta

SERVES 2

PREP: 15 MINUTES

COOK: 2–4 MINUTES

4 thin slices of ciabatta
(about 15g each)
1 garlic clove, halved

**FOR THE TOMATO
AND BASIL TOPPING**

3 ripe tomatoes
10g fresh basil,
leaves shredded
1 tbsp good-quality
extra virgin olive oil
½ garlic clove, very
thinly sliced
flaked sea salt
ground black pepper

**FOR THE MUSHROOM
TOPPING**

15g butter
1 tsp sunflower oil
2 garlic cloves, thinly sliced
150g baby button
mushrooms, quartered
a few fresh thyme sprigs,
leaves stripped
flaked sea salt
ground black pepper

A traditional Italian antipasto (snack or starter), this bruschetta is crispy and fresh tasting – the perfect food for sharing with friends.

To make the tomato and basil topping, make a shallow cross in the bottom of each tomato and place them in a heatproof bowl. Cover with just-boiled water and leave to stand for about a minute or until the skins loosen and begin to peel back.

Drain the tomatoes in a colander and rinse under cold water until cool enough to handle. Peel off the skins, cut the tomatoes into quarters and scoop out the seeds. Dice the tomato flesh.

Mix the tomatoes with the basil, olive oil and garlic. Season with salt and pepper and set aside while the bread is prepared.

Toast or griddle the bread on both sides, then rub with a little garlic and place on a serving platter. Spoon the topping over the toast.

To make the mushroom topping, heat the butter and oil over a medium heat in a large non-stick frying pan. Add the garlic, mushrooms and thyme and cook for 3 minutes or until the mushrooms have softened and are slightly golden. Do not allow the garlic to burn or it will taste bitter. Season the mixture with a good pinch of salt and plenty of freshly ground pepper.

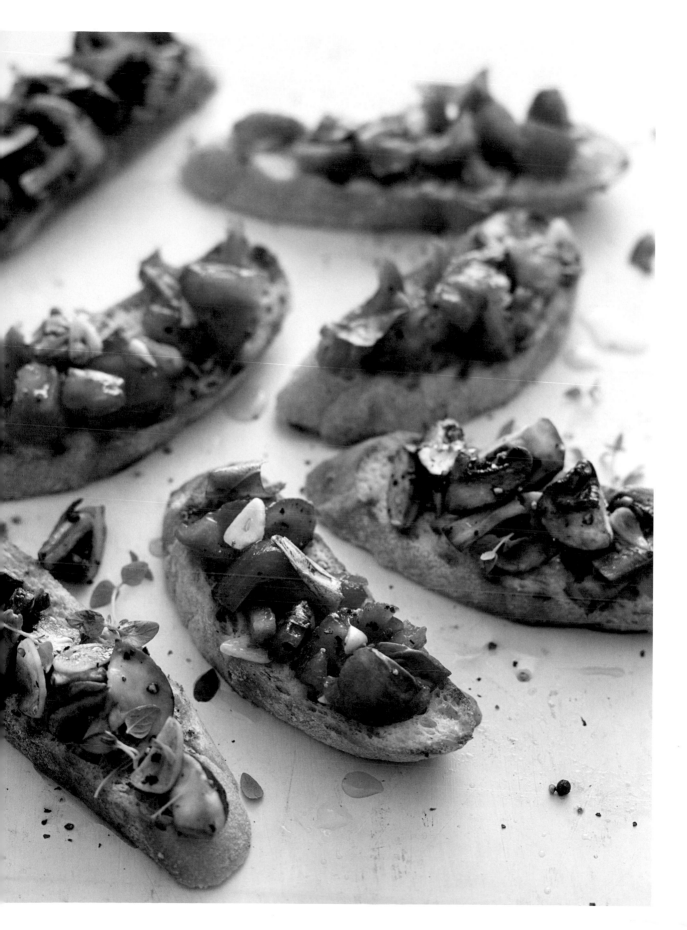

141
CALORIES
PER SERVING

garlic and herb bread

SERVES 6
PREP: 15 MINUTES
COOK: 20 MINUTES

275g ciabatta loaf
    (cut off the ends,
    leaving 200g bread)
40g softened butter
2 small garlic cloves,
    crushed
10g flat-leaf parsley,
    leaves finely chopped
ground black pepper

Freeze the buttered and reassembled (but unbaked) loaf by wrapping tightly in foil. Seal in a freezer-proof bag and freeze for up to 2 months. Bake from frozen, adding 5 minutes to the first baking time.

Everyone's favourite, but make sure you keep track of how many slices you have!

Preheat the oven to 220°C/Fan 200°C/Gas 7. Put the ciabatta on a board and cut it into 18 diagonal slices. Place the bread slices on a large sheet of foil.

Cream the butter, garlic, herbs and a couple of twists of ground black pepper together in a bowl, then spread the mixture over one side of each slice of bread. Assemble the bread back into the shape of the original ciabatta loaf and then loosely wrap the foil around it. Place on a baking tray.

Bake in the oven for 10 minutes or until the bread is hot. Remove it from the oven, carefully open up the foil so the bread is exposed, then return to the oven for a further 8–10 minutes or until golden.

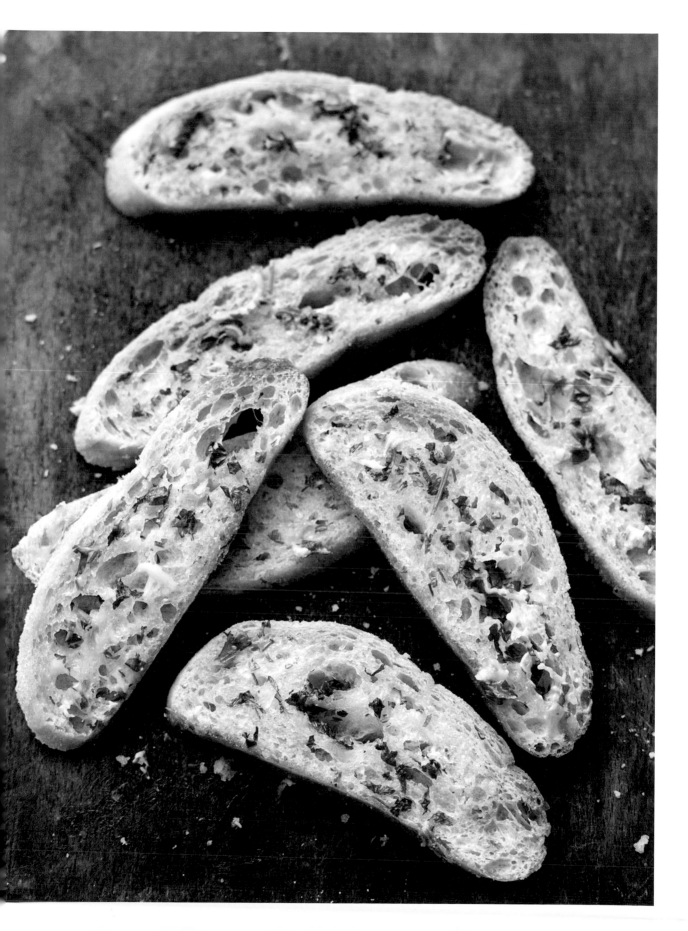

337
CALORIES
PER SERVING

pizza pronto

SERVES 2
PREP: 15 MINUTES
COOK: 3–5 MINUTES

400g can chopped
    tomatoes with herbs
2 tbsp tomato purée
2 large flour tortilla wraps
    (each about 60g)
45g prosciutto or
    wafer-thin ham
20g thinly sliced, ready
    to eat chorizo or
    salami, halved
30g grated mozzarella
30g pitted black or green
    olives (drained)
30g sun-blush (semi-dried)
    tomatoes in oil,
    drained well
ground black pepper

As the name suggests, this is a very quick way to throw together a pizza. It has all the traditional flavours of a deep dish but with less than half the calories. Garnish with fresh basil if you like.

Preheat the grill to its hottest setting and place a large baking tray under the grill to warm. Drain the tomatoes in a sieve until most of the excess juice is gone, tip into a bowl and mix with the tomato purée.

Place one of the tortillas on a chopping board and spread with half of the tomatoes, leaving a 2cm gap around the edges.

Tear the prosciutto or ham into strips and arrange on top of the tomatoes. Add the chorizo or salami, sprinkle with the cheese and season with ground black pepper and chilli flakes.

Slide the pizza from the chopping board onto the preheated baking tray. Place under the hot grill and cook for $1\frac{1}{2}$–$2\frac{1}{2}$ minutes or until the cheese has melted and the edges of the pizza are beginning to brown.

Slide the pizza onto a board or warmed plate and serve immediately. Continue to make the other pizzas in the same way.

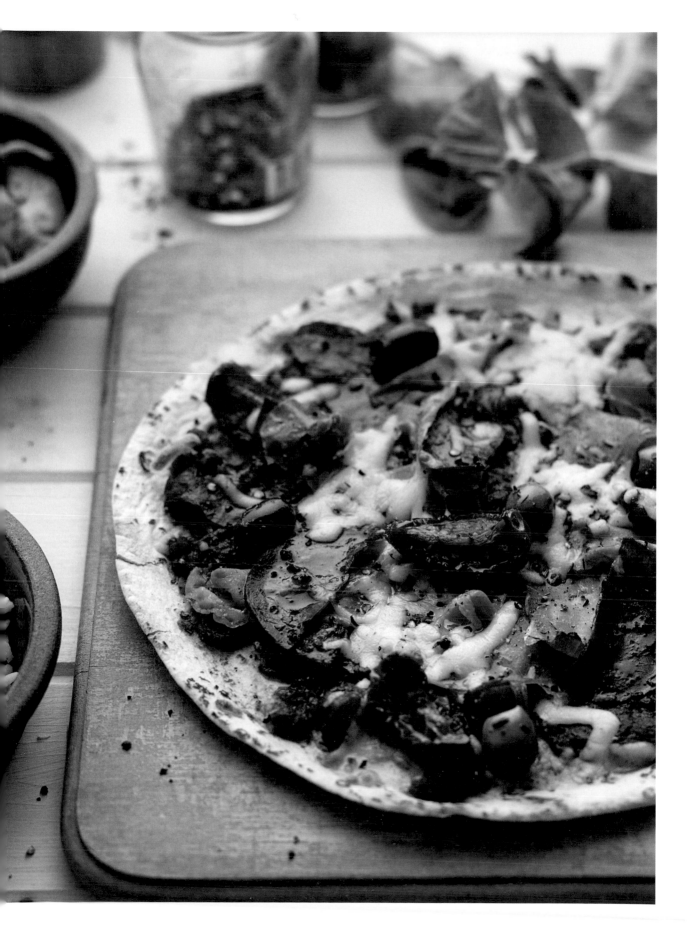

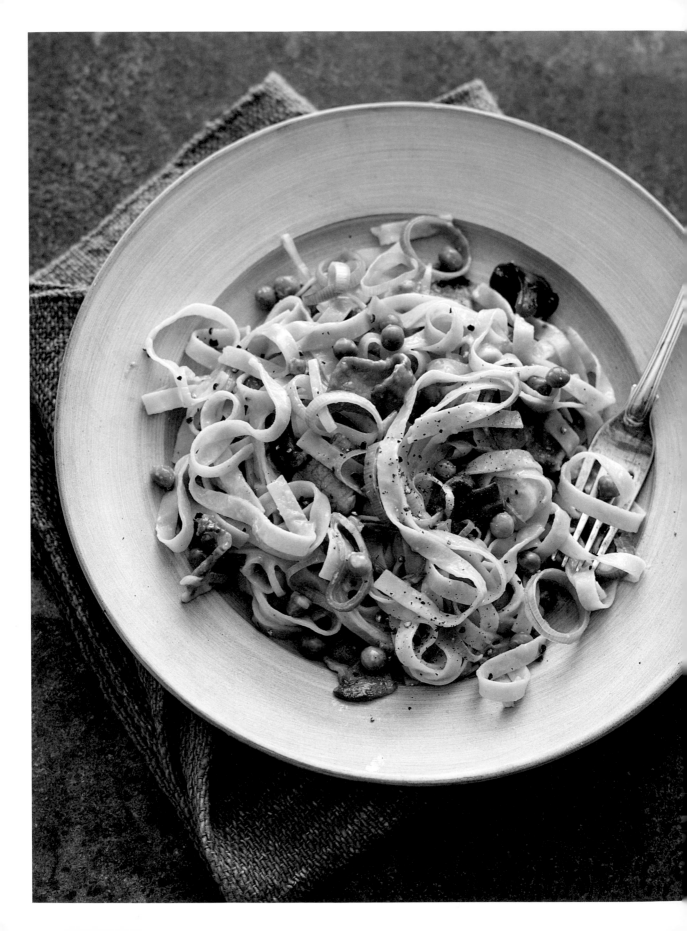

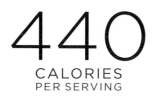

440
CALORIES
PER SERVING

creamy pasta carbonara

SERVES 4
PREP: 15 MINUTES
COOK: 12–15 MINUTES

200g dried tagliatelle
100g frozen peas
oil, for spraying or brushing
4 smoked back bacon
   rashers
150g button mushrooms,
   halved
2 slender leeks, trimmed
   and thinly sliced
2 large eggs, beaten
50g Parmesan cheese,
   finely grated
50ml double cream
flaked sea salt
ground black pepper

This carbonara has all of the traditional tastes and makes a filling and easy supper. The drop of cream is really worth it for the extra richness.

Half fill a large saucepan with water and bring it to the boil. Tip the pasta into the boiling water and cook for 10–12 minutes or according to packet instructions until tender. Add the frozen peas for the last 2 minutes of the cooking time.

Meanwhile, trim the bacon of any visible fat and cut it into 1cm-wide strips. Spray or brush a large non-stick frying pan or wok with oil and place it over a high heat. Add the bacon and mushrooms, season well with salt and pepper and stir-fry for 3–4 minutes. Add the leeks and stir-fry for a further 3 minutes until tender.

Beat the eggs, cheese and cream together in a bowl. Reserve 3 ladlefuls of the pasta cooking water, then drain the pasta in a colander and return it to the pan.

Add the bacon, mushrooms and leeks to the pasta and 2 tablespoons of the reserved cooking water. Pour over the egg mixture and toss together well over a low heat for about a minute or until the egg is hot and creamy. Don't allow it to overheat or the eggs will scramble. Tip the pasta into a warmed serving dish, season with more black pepper and take to the table.

498
CALORIES
PER SERVING

pollo pasta with pesto

SERVES 4
PREP: 15 MINUTES
COOK: 10–15 MINUTES

250g dried pasta, penne,
   twists (fusilli) or spirals
   (cavatappi)
oil, for spraying or brushing
2 boneless, skinless
   chicken breasts
150g button mushrooms,
   quartered
50g sundried tomatoes,
   drained and cut into
   thin strips
4 tbsp fresh basil pesto
50ml single cream
   (optional)
flaked sea salt
ground black pepper

**Easy and packed with flavour, this is a very hearty pasta dish
with just a hint of pesto. It's perfect if you're in need of a quick
family dinner.**

Half fill a large saucepan with water and bring to the boil.
Tip the pasta into the boiling water and cook for 10–12 minutes
or follow the packet instructions until tender. Cut the chicken
into roughly 2.5cm chunks.

Meanwhile, spray or brush a large non-stick frying pan or
wok with oil and place over a high heat. Season the chicken
well with salt and pepper and stir-fry with the mushrooms for
3–4 minutes or until lightly browned. Add the tomatoes and
stir-fry for a further 2 minutes. Remove from the heat.

Drain the pasta in a colander and return to the pan. Add the
chicken mixture and stir in the pesto and cream, if using. Toss
together over a medium heat until the sauce is hot. Season
with more pepper and serve.

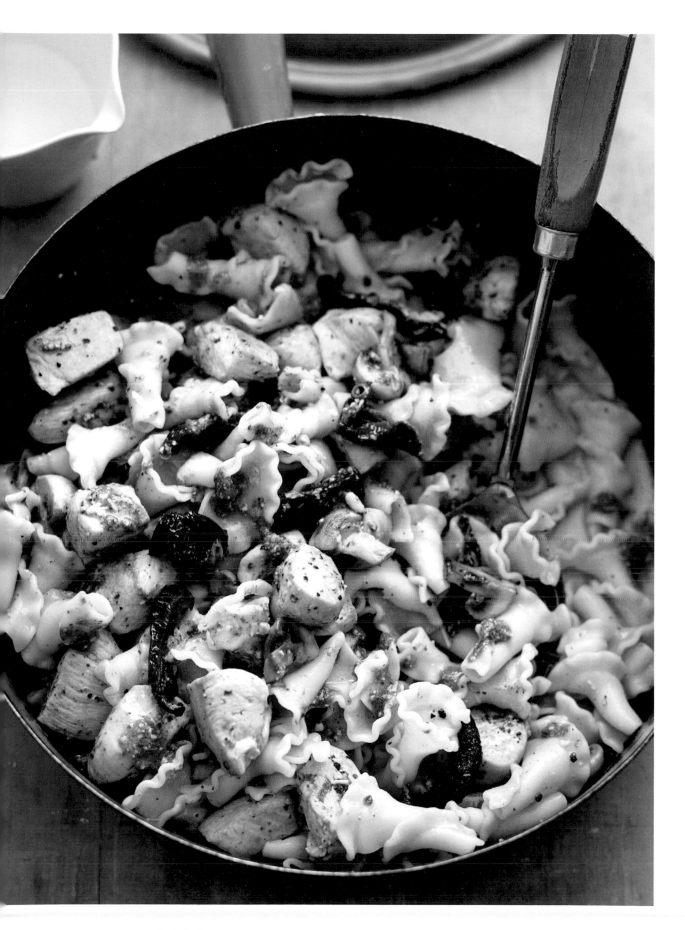

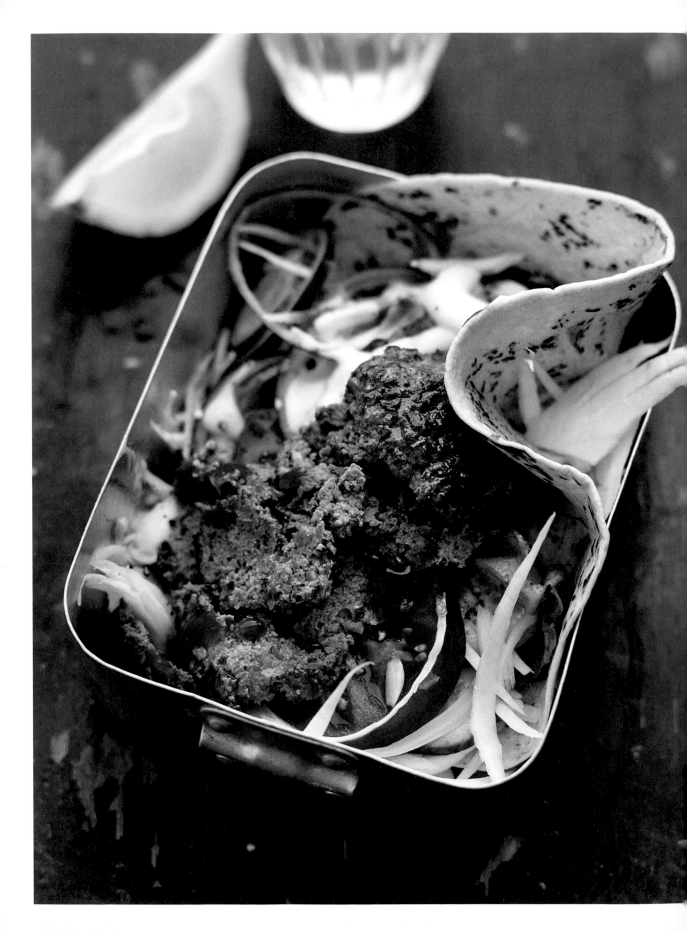

298
CALORIES
PER SERVING

lamb doner kebabs

SERVES 4
PREP: 20 MINUTES
COOK: 40–45 MINUTES,
PLUS RESTING TIME

175g lean lamb leg steaks
   (about 2 steaks)
200g lean minced lamb
½ medium onion,
   roughly chopped
2 garlic cloves, crushed
1½ tsp ground coriander
1½ tsp ground cumin
1 tsp flaked sea salt
oil, for spraying or brushing
4 regular tortilla wraps
   (each about 40g)
ground black pepper

GARLIC SAUCE
3 tbsp fat-free
   natural yoghurt
1 tbsp light mayonnaise
1 garlic clove, crushed
pinch of flaked sea salt

TO SERVE
lettuce, shredded
tomatoes, thinly sliced
cucumber, thinly sliced
white cabbage,
   finely shredded
red onion, cut into rings
lemon wedges,
   for squeezing
hot chilli sauce (optional)

A little different from what you'll find in your local takeaway, I've tried to pack as much flavour into these 'kebabs' as possible. Make sure you get the meat mixture as smooth as possible as it makes the kebab meat taste more authentic.

Preheat the oven to 200°C/Fan 180°C/Gas 6. Trim the lamb steaks, removing any visible fat and cut it into roughly 3cm chunks. Put the lamb mince and steaks in a food processor with the onion, garlic, coriander, cumin, salt and lots of black pepper.

Blitz until as smooth as possible. You may need to remove the lid and push the mixture down a couple of times until the right consistency is reached.

Put the lamb mixture in a greased roasting tin and form it into a loaf shape, roughly 14 x 7cm and 5cm high. Cook in the oven for 40–45 minutes or until well browned and cooked through.

Meanwhile, make the garlic sauce. Mix all the ingredients in a small bowl and set aside.

Leave the lamb to rest for 5 minutes. Warm the tortillas in the hot oven for 1–2 minutes. Using a sharp knife, carefully shave the rested lamb diagonally into thin slices.

Fill the warmed tortillas with salad and the hot lamb and season with black pepper. Spoon over the garlic sauce, add a squeeze of lemon and some hot chilli sauce too if you like.

419

CALORIES
PER SERVING

chicken shish kebab

SERVES 4
PREP: 10 MINUTES,
PLUS MARINATING TIME
COOK: 10–12 MINUTES

3 boneless, skinless
    chicken breasts
oil, for brushing
4 large tortilla wraps
    or flatbreads (each
    about 60g)
lemon wedges, for squeezing

FOR THE MARINADE
4 tbsp fresh lemon juice
2 garlic cloves, crushed
$\frac{1}{2}$ tsp cayenne pepper
1 tsp ground cumin
1 tbsp olive oil
$\frac{1}{2}$ flaked sea salt
1 tsp ground black pepper

FOR THE GREEK SALAD
$\frac{1}{2}$ medium red onion
$\frac{1}{2}$ tsp dried oregano
2 tbsp red wine vinegar
3 large ripe tomatoes
1 cucumber
50g feta cheese, cut
    into small cubes
50g pitted black
    olives, drained
small handful fresh
    mint leaves
2 tsp extra virgin olive oil
flaked sea salt
ground black pepper

Freeze the raw, marinated
chicken pieces in a zip-seal
bag for up to 2 months.
Thaw in the fridge overnight
and cook as the recipe. The
Greek salad is unsuitable
for freezing.

**This kebab is better than anything you could get at the local
takeaway – it's straight off the grill, juicy and full of flavour.
If you serve the chicken and salad without the wrap, you
will save around 185 calories per serving.**

Cut the chicken into 2.5cm cubes and put it in a large non-
metallic bowl. Add all the marinade ingredients, and stir well.
Cover and leave to marinate for 1–4 hours in the fridge.

To make the salad, slice the onion thinly and put it in a medium
bowl. Stir in the oregano and vinegar and leave to stand for
30 minutes. Cut the tomatoes into 6–8 wedges, then cut each
wedge in half. Add the tomatoes to the bowl with the onion.
Season well with salt and pepper. Trim the cucumber and cut
it into chunky pieces. Toss the cucumber, feta, olives and
mint leaves with the onion and tomatoes. Pour over the oil
and set aside.

Preheat a griddle over a high heat or set the grill to its hottest
setting. Push the chicken pieces onto 4 long metal skewers,
squashing the chicken fairly closely together. Brush the griddle
lightly with oil and cook the chicken for 10–12 minutes, turning
every now and then, until cooked through and lightly charred.

Alternatively, grill on a rack over a foil-lined baking tray
for about 10 minutes, turning occasionally, until cooked
throughout. Heat the wraps on the griddle or under the grill.

Divide the salad and wraps between plates and top with
the chicken. Serve with lemon wedges for squeezing over.

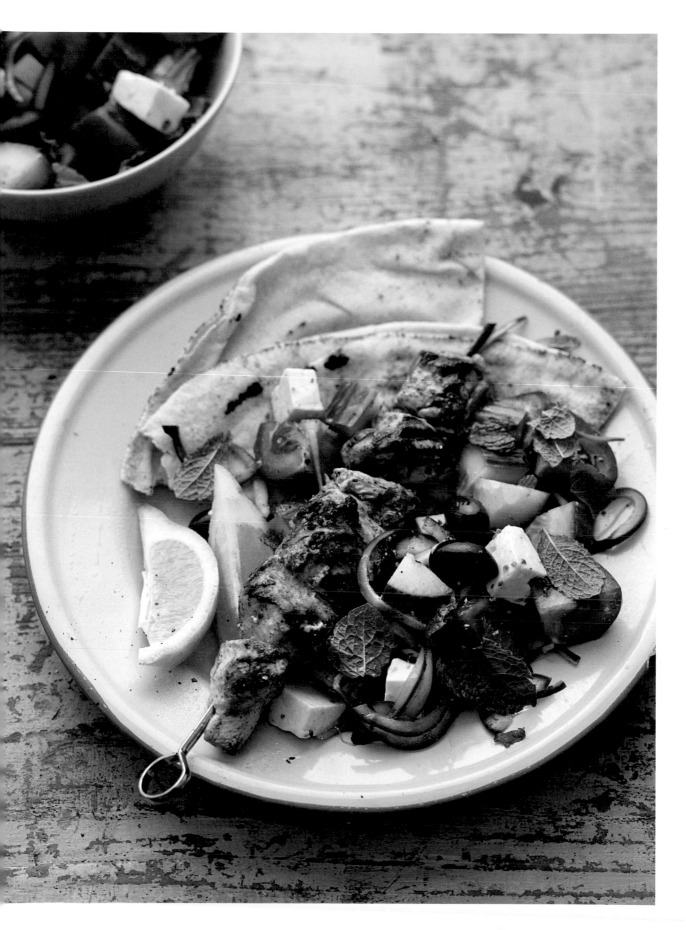

344
CALORIES
PER SERVING

stifado

SERVES 6
PREP: 20–30 MINUTES
COOK: 2 HOURS

1.2kg braising beef
   (such as chuck steak)
1 tbsp olive oil
400g shallots (about 24),
   peeled
1 tsp fennel seeds
2 bay leaves
1 cinnamon stick
3 bushy fresh thyme sprigs
1 fresh rosemary stalk
3 tbsp red wine vinegar
200ml red wine
400g can chopped
   tomatoes
200ml beef stock (made
   with 1 beef stock cube)
roughly chopped flat-leaf
   parsley, to garnish
   (optional)
flaked sea salt
ground black pepper

Freeze the cooled stew
in zip-seal bags or in
freezer-proof containers
for up to 4 months. Thaw in
the fridge overnight. Reheat
thoroughly in a large, wide-
based saucepan, stirring
gently until piping hot.

A rich Greek beef stew full of sweet shallots. The large pieces of beef do take a while to simmer into tenderness, so plan ahead when making it. Serve with a small portion of rice.

Preheat the oven to 180°C/Fan 160°C/Gas 4. Trim the beef of any hard fat or sinew and cut into roughly 4cm chunks. Pour 1 teaspoon of the oil into a large, non-stick frying pan and place over a high heat. Season the beef and add it to the pan. Fry in two batches, adding another teaspoon of oil for the second batch, for 2–3 minutes each or until the beef is browned, turning every now and then. Transfer the beef to a flameproof casserole.

Return the frying pan to the heat with the remaining oil. Fry the shallots for 5 minutes, turning often, until browned on all sides. Add the fennel seeds, bay leaves, cinnamon, thyme and rosemary and fry for a few seconds, while stirring. Take off the heat. Deglaze the pan with the vinegar and pour all the shallots, spices and herbs over the beef in the casserole.

Stir in the red wine, tomatoes and beef stock. Bring to a simmer. Cover the surface with a circle of baking parchment, so the beef is kept moist, then pop a lid on top and transfer to the oven.

Cook for 1¾ hours or until the beef is very tender – test a piece by cutting it in half with a sharp knife. If it remains fairly firm, return the dish to the oven and continue cooking for a further 30 minutes or until tender. Scatter with roughly chopped parsley before serving if you like.

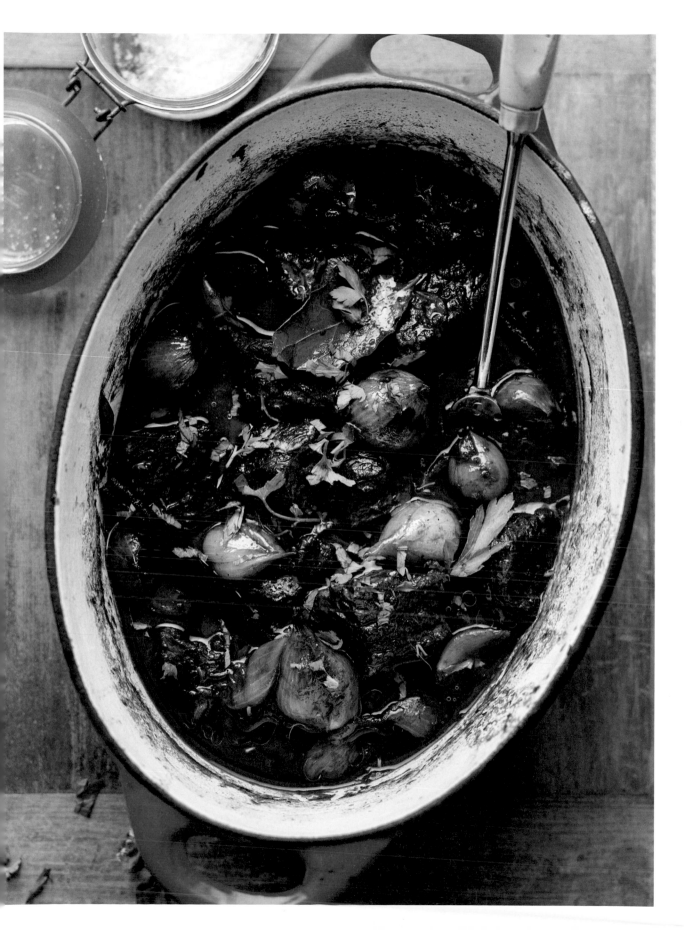

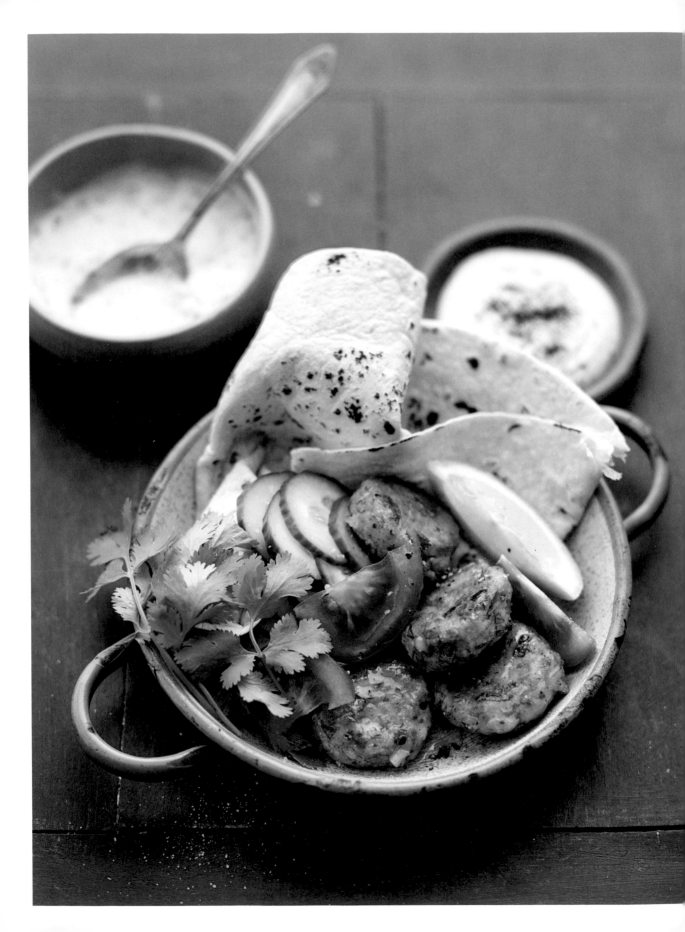

260
CALORIES
PER SERVING

falafel

SERVES 4
PREP: 20 MINUTES
COOK: 8–12 MINUTES

1½ tsp cumin seeds
1 tsp coriander seeds
3 garlic cloves, peeled
1 tsp flaked sea salt
400g can chickpeas,
    drained and rinsed
½ medium onion,
    coarsely grated
20g fresh coriander,
    leaves roughly chopped,
    plus extra to garnish
20g fresh flat-leaf parsley,
    leaves roughly chopped
50g plain flour
1 egg yolk, beaten
2 tsp sunflower oil
ground black pepper
4 regular tortilla wraps
    (each about 40g),
    warmed
minted yoghurt sauce
    (see page 40)

TO SERVE
cucumber, thinly sliced
tomato, cut into wedges
lemon wedges,
    for squeezing

Open freeze the cooked
falafel until solid before
transferring them to a
freezer-proof container.
Cover, label and freeze for
up to 3 months. To defrost,
thaw and warm in a low
oven or microwave briefly.
The yoghurt sauce is not
suitable for freezing.

These falafel make a really good addition to any picnic or
packed lunch and can be eaten hot or cold. For some extra
heat, add a dribble of hot chilli sauce. Serve with salad and
minted yoghurt sauce (see page 40).

Start by making the minted yoghurt sauce on page 40.
Cover and chill until needed.

Put the cumin and coriander seeds in a pestle and mortar
and pound until crushed to a powder. Add the garlic and
salt and pound to a paste. Scrape everything into a food
processor and add the chickpeas, onion and lots of black
pepper. Blitz to a thick, slightly crunchy mixture. It shouldn't
be too smooth as you are looking for some texture to give
the falafel a bit of bite.

Transfer the mixture to a mixing bowl and stir in the herbs,
flour and egg yolk. Mix with clean hands until thoroughly
combined. Form the mixture into 16 walnut-sized balls
and flatten slightly.

Pour 1 teaspoon of the oil into a large non-stick frying pan
and place over a medium heat. Fry the falafel in two batches
for 2–3 minutes on each side or until nicely browned and hot
throughout, adding another teaspoon of oil after the first
batch is cooked.

Serve the hot falafel with warmed wraps, cucumber, tomato,
lemon wedges for squeezing and minted yoghurt sauce.

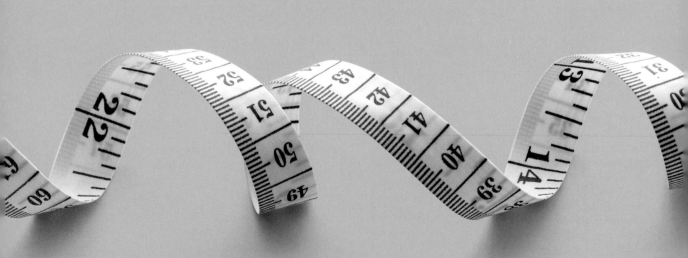

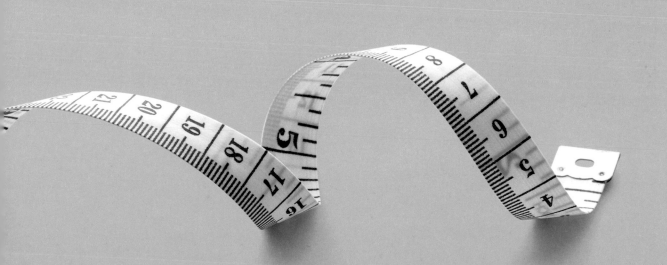

usa

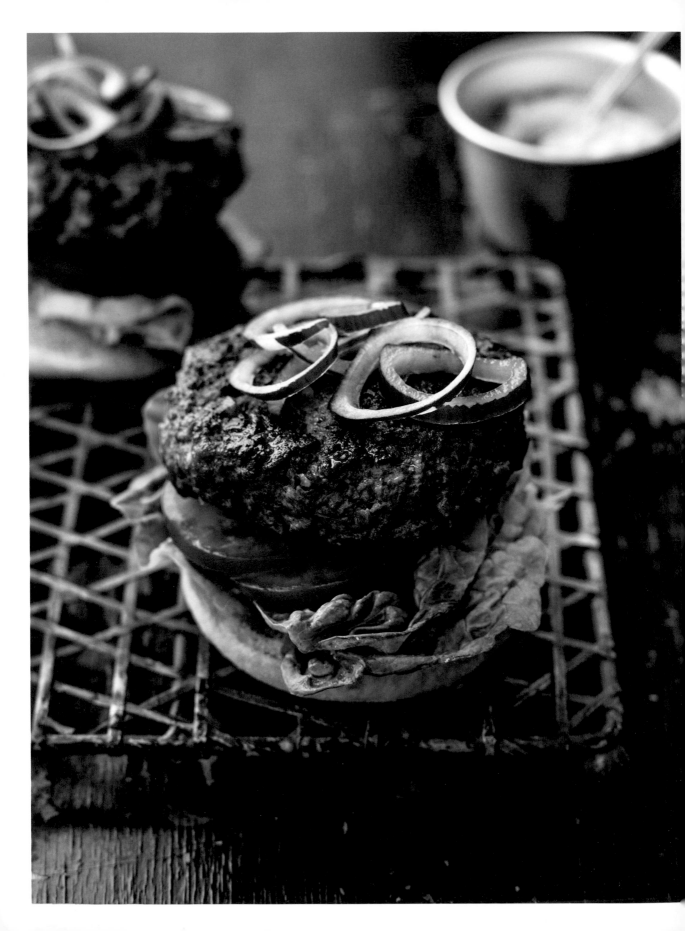

342
CALORIES
PER SERVING

lower fat burgers

SERVES 4
PREP: 15 MINUTES
COOK: 10–12 MINUTES

500g lean beef mince
1 medium onion,
  coarsely grated
1 large carrot, peeled
  and finely grated
2 garlic cloves, crushed
1 heaped tsp dried
  mixed herbs
oil, for spraying or brushing
2 English muffins
flaked sea salt
ground black pepper

TO SERVE
baby gem lettuce leaves
tomatoes, thinly sliced
red onion, thinly sliced

Freeze the individually foil
wrapped and uncooked
burgers in a zip-seal bag
for up to 2 months. Thaw
overnight in the fridge
before following the
cooking instructions
as the recipe.

Tip: Mix light mayonnaise
with a little harissa paste
for a spicy sauce to serve
with the burgers.

These burgers use a smart trick that not only keeps the meat deliciously juicy but also sneaks in some vegetables that some picky eaters might otherwise avoid. Serve with oven-baked chips (see below) if you like.

Put the mince in a large bowl with the onion, carrot, garlic and herbs. Add a good pinch of salt and plenty of black pepper. Mix until well combined – you can use clean hands for this if you like. Form the mixture into four balls and flatten into burger shapes.

Spray or brush a large non-stick frying pan with oil and fry the burgers gently for 5–6 minutes on each side or until nicely browned and cooked through.

Cut the English muffins in half and toast. Serve a burger on each muffin with lettuce, tomato and red onion. Accompany with oven-baked chips (see below).

Oven-baked chips: Preheat the oven to 220°C/Fan 200°C/Gas 7. Half fill a large saucepan with water and bring to the boil. Peel 600g potatoes and cut into chips. Carefully add the chips to the water and return to the boil. Par-boil the chips for 4 minutes then drain well in a colander. While still in the colander, spray the chips with oil and toss a few times until lightly coated. Scatter the chips over a baking tray and season with salt and lots of black pepper. Bake for 20 minutes then turn with a spatula. Spray with more oil and return to the oven for a further 10 minutes until golden and crisp. Serves 4. Calories per serving: 119

190
CALORIES
PER SERVING

spicy bean burgers

SERVES 4
PREP: 15 MINUTES
COOK: 25–30 MINUTES

oil, for spraying
1 medium red onion,
    finely chopped
2 garlic cloves, crushed
2 tbsp chipotle paste
    (from a jar)
4 tbsp fresh white
    breadcrumbs
400g can chickpeas,
    drained and rinsed
400g can red kidney beans,
    drained and rinsed
20g fresh coriander,
    leaves finely chopped
finely grated zest of 1 lime
flaked sea salt
freshly ground black pepper

TO SERVE
tomatoes, finely sliced
baby gem lettuce leaves
lime wedges

Open freeze the unbaked
burgers on a parchment
lined tray until solid. Pack
the burgers into a freezer-
proof container and freeze
for up to 3 months. Cook
from frozen as the recipe,
adding an extra 5–10
minutes until hot
throughout.

Crisp on the outside, with a decidedly Tex Mex chipotle twist on the inside, these veggie burgers are full of flavour. Forming the burgers can be a messy job; I've found that using wet hands can help.

Preheat the oven to 220°C/Fan 200°C/Gas 7.

Spray a large frying pan with oil and place over a medium heat. Fry the onion and garlic for about 3 minutes until soft, stirring regularly. Cool for 5 minutes.

Transfer the fried onion and garlic to a food processor and add the chipotle paste, breadcrumbs and half each of the chickpeas and beans. Season with a good pinch of salt and some black pepper. Blitz until as smooth as possible. You may need to push the mixture down with a rubber spatula a few times until the right consistency is reached.

Add the remaining chickpeas and beans, the coriander and lime zest and pulse a few times until combined but not totally smooth. Form the mixture into eight balls and flatten to about 2cm thick.

Spray or brush a large baking tray with oil and lay the burgers on top. Bake for 20–25 minutes, turning halfway through the cooking time. The burgers should be crisp on the outside and hot throughout.

Serve stacked on a slice of tomato, with plenty of fresh green salad, lime and coriander mayo (see below) and lime wedges for squeezing.

Lime and coriander mayo: Mix 4 tablespoons light mayonnaise with 4 tablespoons soured cream, 1 tablespoon fresh lime juice and 2 tablespoons fresh coriander. Serves 4. Calories per serving: 45

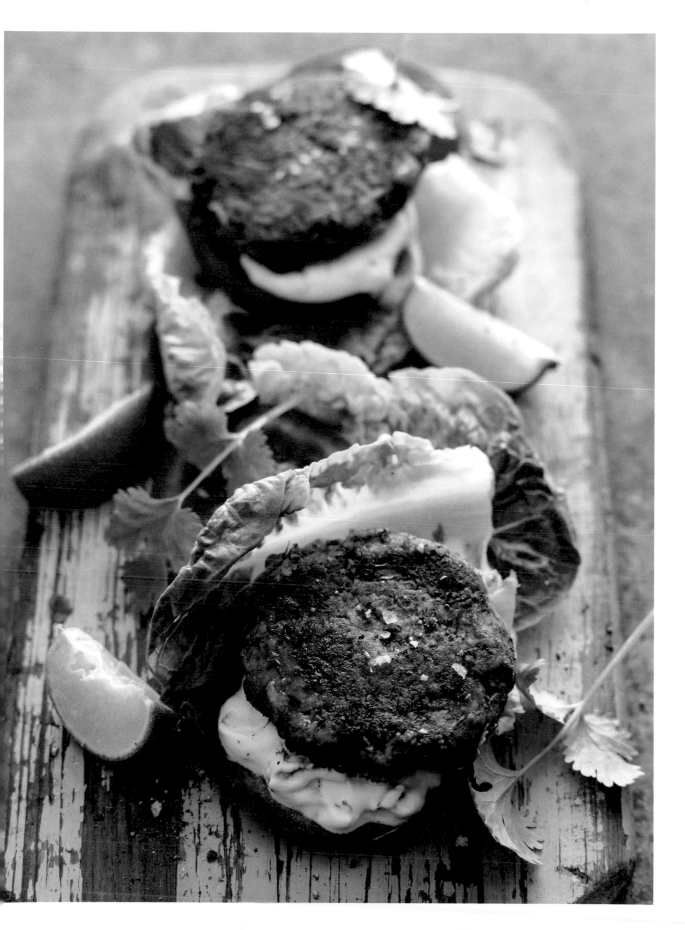

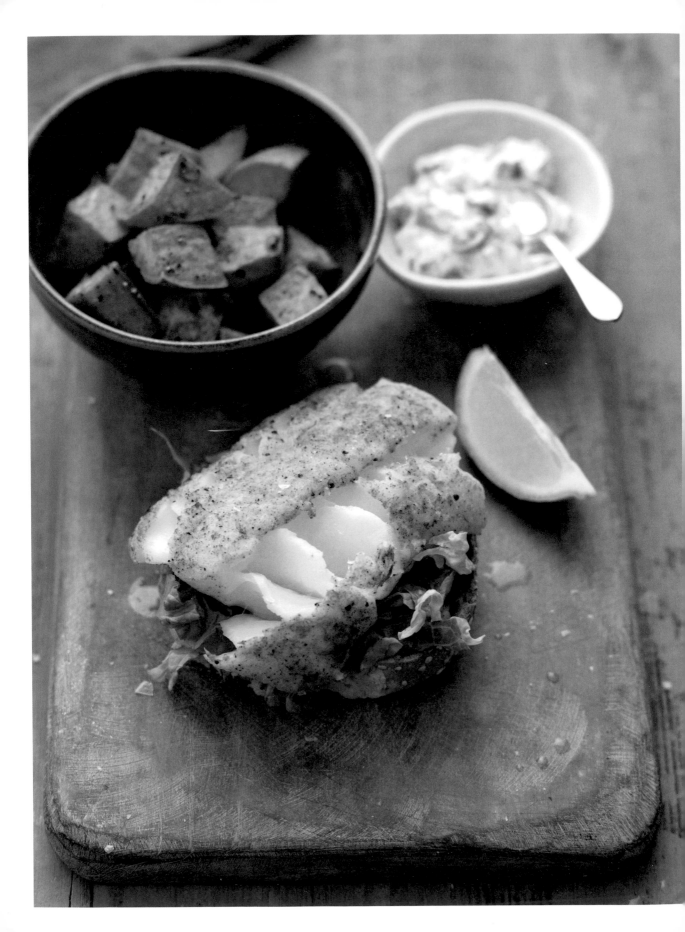

270
CALORIES
PER SERVING

fish burgers
with tartare sauce

SERVES 4
PREP: 15 MINUTES
COOK: 6 MINUTES

4 tbsp plain flour
½ tsp paprika (not smoked)
¼ tsp hot chilli powder
pinch of ground turmeric
1 tsp fine sea salt
½ tsp freshly ground
    black pepper
4 thick, skinless white fish
    fillets, such as cod or
    haddock (each about 150g)
oil, for spraying or brushing
2 burger buns

TO SERVE
lettuce, shredded
tomatoes, sliced
lemon wedges,
    for squeezing
tartare sauce (see right)

Fresh, crispy and surprisingly easy to prepare; these burgers make a nice change from soggy fish-finger sandwiches. A small portion of baked sweet potato chunks goes well and will add an extra 137 calories per each 150g (raw weight) portion.

Mix the flour with the paprika, chilli powder, turmeric, salt and pepper. Put half the flour in a large freezer bag.

Take a fish fillet and drop it into the bag. Toss until lightly coated, then transfer the fillet to a large baking tray lined with non-stick baking paper. Do the same with a second fillet, then add the rest of the seasoned flour to the bag and coat the remaining fish fillets in exactly the same way.

Spray or brush a large frying pan with oil and fry the fish for 2½–3½ minutes on each side or until golden brown and cooked through. If your fillets are particularly thick, finish cooking them in a moderate oven.

Cut the burger buns in half and arrange, cut-side up, on 4 plates (half a bun per serving). Top with the lettuce, tomatoes and tartare sauce. Put the fish fillets on top, add lemon wedges for squeezing and serve.

Tartare sauce: Mix 2 tablespoons light mayonnaise, 2 tablespoons fat-free natural yoghurt and 1 teaspoon Dijon mustard in a bowl. Stir in 50g drained and roughly chopped capers, 50g drained and thinly sliced mini gherkins (cornichons), 2 tablespoons finely chopped fresh curly parsley leaves, 1 tablespoon finely chopped fresh tarragon leaves and plenty of ground black pepper. Adjust the salt if necessary. Cover the surface of the sauce with cling film and stand for at least 20 minutes to allow the flavours to mingle. Serves 4. Calories per serving: 34

352
CALORIES
PER SERVING

southern-style chicken

SERVES 4
PREP: 20 MINUTES
COOK: 25–30 MINUTES

12 boneless, skinless chicken
   thighs (about 1kg)
150ml reduced-fat
   evaporated milk
1 tbsp Worcestershire sauce
75g plain flour
1½ tsp dried thyme
1 tbsp paprika (not smoked)
½ tsp hot chilli powder
1 tsp flaked sea salt
oil, for spraying
ground black pepper

Open freeze the uncooked
but coated chicken thighs
then pack them into a
freezer-proof container,
interleaving them with
baking parchment. Freeze
for up to 3 months. Cook
from frozen as the recipe,
increasing the cooking time
by 12–15 minutes or until
the chicken is cooked and
piping hot throughout.

**This chicken is so delicious that no one will guess that it
is low-fat. I've used boneless, skinless chicken thighs and
trimmed off as much fat as possible, which could save
around 100 calories per portion!**

Preheat the oven to 220°C/Fan 200°C/Gas 7. Trim all visible
fat from the chicken thighs so they are as lean as possible.

Pour the evaporated milk into a bowl and add the
Worcestershire sauce. Put the flour, thyme, paprika, chilli
powder, salt and plenty of freshly ground black pepper
in a separate bowl and mix thoroughly.

Transfer half of the seasoned flour to a large, shallow bowl.
One at a time, dip the chicken thighs in the evaporated milk,
then into the seasoned flour and turn until evenly coated. Shake
off any excess. Place them on a baking tray lined with baking
parchment. After you have coated 6 thighs, put the rest of the
seasoned flour in the bowl and continue tossing the remaining
chicken. Once all the chicken is on the tray, spray evenly with
the cooking oil, ensuring all the seasoning is lightly coated.

Bake the chicken for 25–30 minutes or until golden brown
and cooked through.

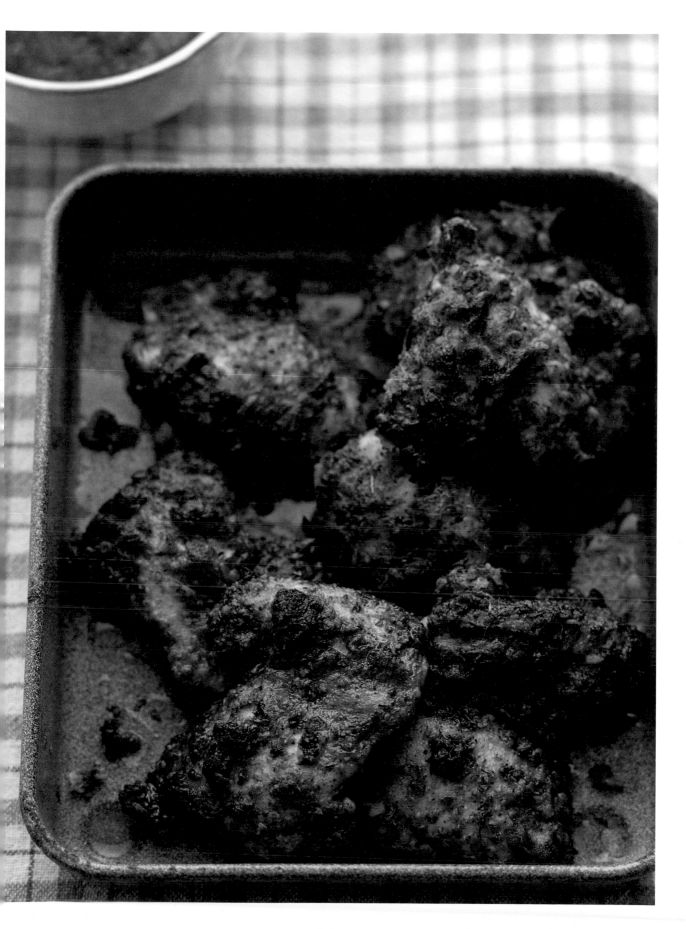

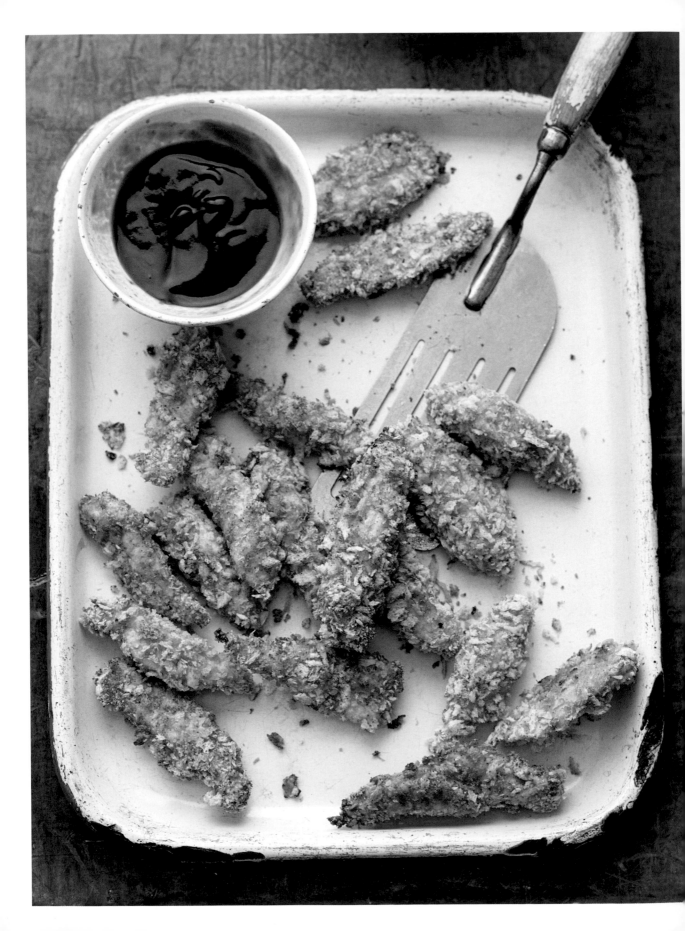

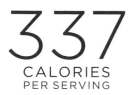

337
CALORIES
PER SERVING

crispy chicken strips

SERVES 4

**PREP: 20 MINUTES,
PLUS CHILLING TIME**

COOK: 15 MINUTES

4 boneless, skinless
   chicken breasts
40g plain flour
½ tsp paprika
   (not smoked)
1 large egg
100g dry white coarse
   breadcrumbs or Japanese
   panko breadcrumbs
oil, for spraying
flaked sea salt
ground black pepper

Open freeze the uncooked
but coated chicken pieces,
then pack them into a
freezer-proof container,
interleaving them with
baking parchment. Freeze
for up to 3 months. Cook
from frozen as the recipe,
increasing the cooking
time by 5–10 minutes or
until the chicken is piping
hot throughout.

**These little chicken strips freeze beautifully and only take
20–25 minutes to cook from frozen. It is well worth having
a big batch on standby!**

Put the chicken breasts on a board and cut each piece into
thin slices at a slight diagonal angle from one end to the other.

Sift the flour and paprika onto a large plate and season with
salt and pepper. Beat the egg in a bowl with a metal whisk
until smooth. Sprinkle half the breadcrumbs into a large bowl.

Take the chicken breast pieces, one at a time, and dust them
in the flour. Shake off any excess, dip them straight into the
beaten egg and then coat them in the breadcrumbs until evenly
covered. Put each piece on a tray lined with baking parchment
while the rest are prepared, adding the reserved breadcrumbs
to the large bowl after coating roughly half the chicken pieces.

Preheat the oven to 200°C/Fan 180°C/Gas 6. Take the chicken
out of the fridge and mist with the oil. Bake in the oven for 15
minutes until the chicken is crisp, golden brown and cooked
through. There should be no pinkness remaining in the centre.

354

CALORIES
PER SERVING

smoky pulled pork

SERVES 6

**PREP: 15 MINUTES,
PLUS MARINATING TIME**

COOK: 4½–5½ HOURS

1.2kg boneless
    shoulder pork
150ml cold water

DRY SPICE RUB
25g soft dark brown sugar
1 tsp smoked hot paprika
1 tsp flaked sea salt
½ tsp cayenne pepper
1 tsp coarsely ground
    black pepper
1 tsp dry mustard powder

TO SERVE
6 white baps
apple sauce (see below)

Juicy and succulent, pulled pork can be a bit greasy at times, which is why this leaner version is much better for your waistline. I always cook mine with the rind and fat, then carefully remove as much as possible before serving. That way, the pork remains moist during cooking but I can still cut the calories.

To make the spice rub, put all the ingredients in a bowl and mix well. Put the pork on a board and rub all over with the spice mix. Transfer the pork to a shallow dish and cover loosely with cling film. Leave in the fridge for 1 hour.

Preheat the oven to 200°C/Fan 180°C/Gas 6. Stand the pork, fat-side up, on top of two sheets of foil in a roasting tin – the foil needs to be big enough to be wrapped around the pork later. Roast for 30 minutes.

Take the pork out of the oven and pour the water into the tin. Reduce the oven temperature to 140°C/Fan 120°C/Gas 1. Wrap the foil around the pork, pinching around the edges to make a good seal. Put the pork in the oven and cook for 4–5 hours until meltingly soft.

When the pork is cooked, transfer it to a board. Remove the rind and fat and pull the pork into shreds with a couple of forks. Split the baps and fill with the hot pork. Serve with apple sauce (see below) and a large salad.

Apple sauce: Peel 1 Bramley cooking apple (about 250g) and 2 eating apples (about 175g each) and cut into chunky pieces. Put the apples in a non-stick saucepan with 50g light soft brown sugar and ½ teaspoon of ground cinnamon. Add 100ml of water, place the pan over a low heat, cover loosely and cook for 15–20 minutes, stirring regularly until the apples are tender and the sauce is thick. Leave to cool, then spoon into a serving dish. Serves 6. Calories per serving: 66

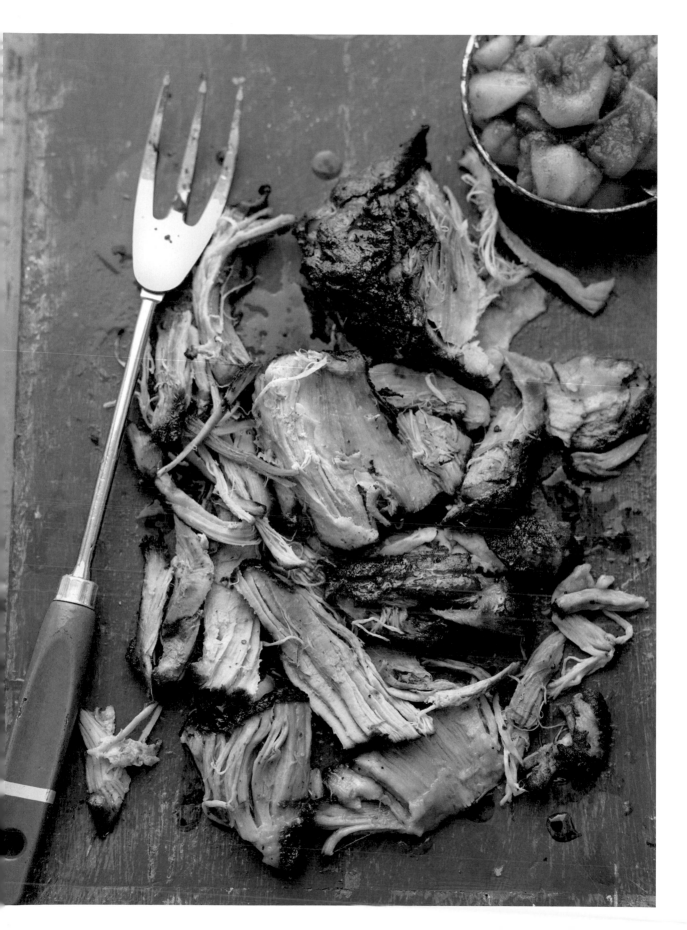

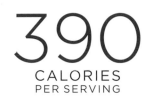

390
CALORIES
PER SERVING

buffalo wings with blue cheese dip

SERVES 4

PREP: 25 MINUTES

COOK: 45 MINUTES

1 tsp sunflower oil,
  for brushing
800g chicken wings
1 tsp hot chilli powder
2 tsp paprika (not smoked)
1 tsp flaked sea salt
coarsely ground
  black pepper
celery sticks, to serve

BASTING SAUCE
5 tbsp ketchup
2 tbsp clear honey
1 tbsp cider vinegar
2 tsp Worcestershire sauce

BLUE CHEESE DIP
50g Stilton cheese
  (or other tangy blue
  cheese), roughly
  crumbled
50g soured cream
50g fat-free natural yoghurt

Freeze the seasoned but
uncooked chicken wings in
large zip-seal bags for up to
4 months. Thaw overnight
in the fridge and follow the
recipe to cook.

A classic American bar snack, great for eating while watching a football match. Serve as a weekend lunch or supper with a big salad on the side. Even if you don't like blue cheese give the dip a go – its tanginess may surprise you and it complements the wings perfectly.

Preheat the oven to 200°C/Fan 180°C/Gas 6. Line a medium baking tray with foil and then brush with oil. Put the chicken wings on a board and cut through the main joint between each part of the wing to give two meaty pieces.

Mix the chilli powder, paprika and some salt and pepper together in a large bowl. Place all the chicken wing pieces in and toss in the seasoning until lightly coated. Scatter the chicken over the baking tray and cook in the centre of the oven for 20 minutes. Turn the chicken with tongs and cook for 15 minutes more.

While the chicken is cooking, make the basting sauce. Put the ketchup, honey, vinegar and Worcestershire sauce in a bowl and stir until thoroughly combined. Take the chicken out of the oven and pour over the sauce. Toss the chicken to coat in the sauce and return to the oven for about 10 minutes, until shiny and glossy.

To make the dip, mash the cheese in a bowl with a fork and mix with the soured cream and yoghurt until almost smooth. (For a smoother sauce, blitz with a stick blender.) Spoon into a serving dish and put it on a platter with celery sticks.

As soon as the chicken is ready, transfer the wings to the platter and serve hot with plenty of napkins!

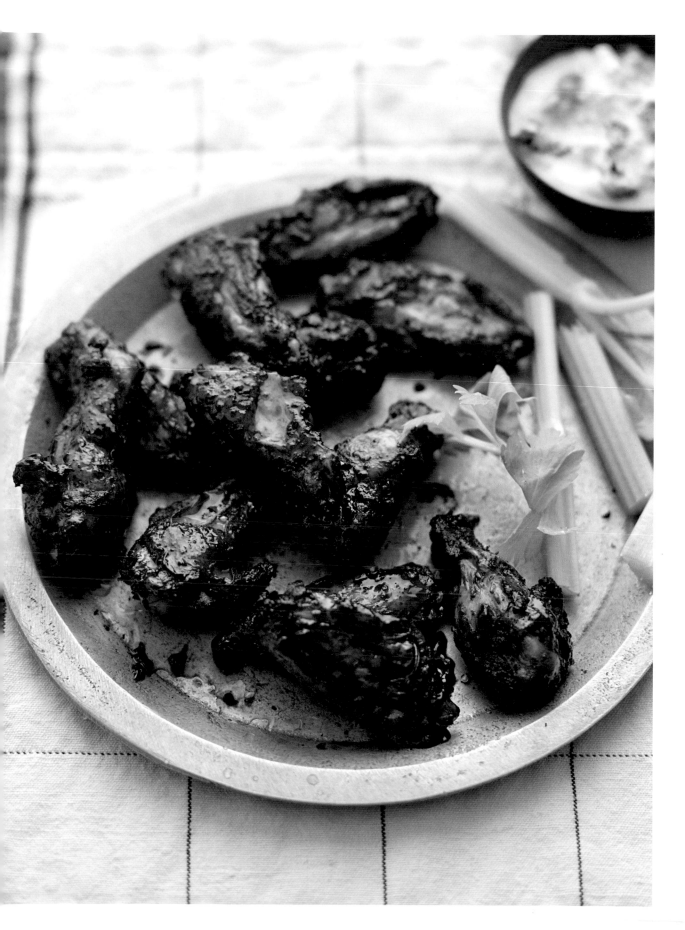

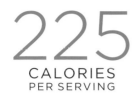

225
CALORIES
PER SERVING

sticky pork 'ribs' in barbecue sauce

SERVES 4
PREP: 10 MINUTES
COOK: 20 MINUTES

4 pork loin steaks
   (each about 170g)
flaked sea salt
ground black pepper

BARBECUE SAUCE
4 tbsp ketchup
2 tbsp clear honey
1 tbsp Worcestershire sauce
½ tsp chilli powder

TO SERVE
coleslaw (see right)
corn on the cob

These 'ribs' are much leaner than a traditional rack of ribs but have all the same flavours. Serve with corn on the cob and the coleslaw suggested below for a true American feast.

Preheat the oven to 200°C/Fan 180°C/Gas 6. To make the barbecue sauce, mix the ingredients together in a bowl and set aside.

Put the pork on a board and trim off any visible fat. Cut the pork into long strips, each around 2cm wide. Season the pork with salt and pepper and place on a foil-lined baking tray. Bake in the oven for 10 minutes. Remove from the oven and carefully drain off any liquid. Coat in the barbecue sauce and return to the oven for 10 minutes or until the sauce is very thick and sticky. Serve with coleslaw (see below) and corn on the cob, if you like. (One medium corn on the cob contains around 75 calories).

Coleslaw: Mix 6 tablespoons fat-free Greek yoghurt and 4 tablespoons light mayonnaise in a large bowl. Finely shred ¼ small white cabbage and ¼ small red cabbage, coarsely grate 1 large carrot and finely slice 4 trimmed spring onions and add them to the bowl. Add 4 tablespoons cold water and season with ground black pepper. Toss together until well combined. Serves 4. Calories per serving: 81

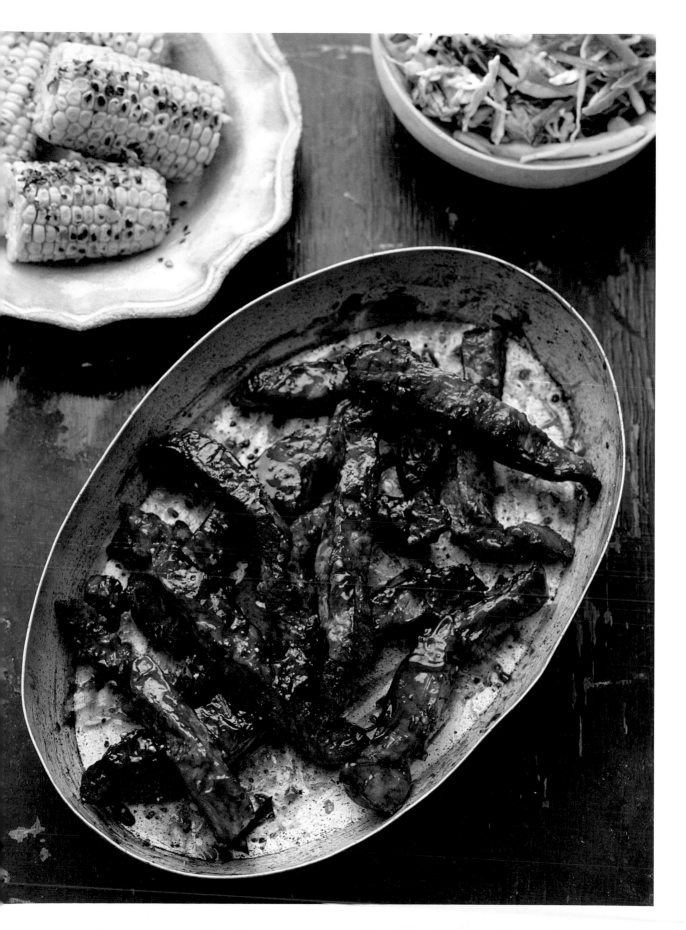

thick strawberry milkshake

SERVES 1
PREP: 10 MINUTES

50g fresh strawberries
150ml semi-skimmed milk
50g vanilla ice cream
3 ice cubes

Tip: Make sure your blender is designed to crush ice or the jug could crack.

Creamy, frothy and sweet; these milkshakes are decadent but light. The ice cream may be a surprising addition but don't worry, the small quantity is definitely worth it and won't do much harm in terms of calories – simply choose an ice cream with 100 calories or less per 100g.

Hull the strawberries by pulling out or cutting off the green leafy bit at the top. Put in a blender with the milk, ice cream and ice cubes. Blitz until smooth and frothy. Pour into a glass and serve.

Chocolate milkshake: Put 1 tablespoon hot chocolate powder, 150ml cold semi-skimmed milk, 50g vanilla ice cream and 3 ice cubes in a blender and blitz until smooth, thick and frothy. Serves 1. Calories per serving: 160

Banana milkshake: Peel and slice 1 very ripe banana and put in a blender with 100ml cold semi-skimmed milk and 3 ice cubes. Blitz until smooth, thick and frothy. Serves 1. Calories per serving: 140

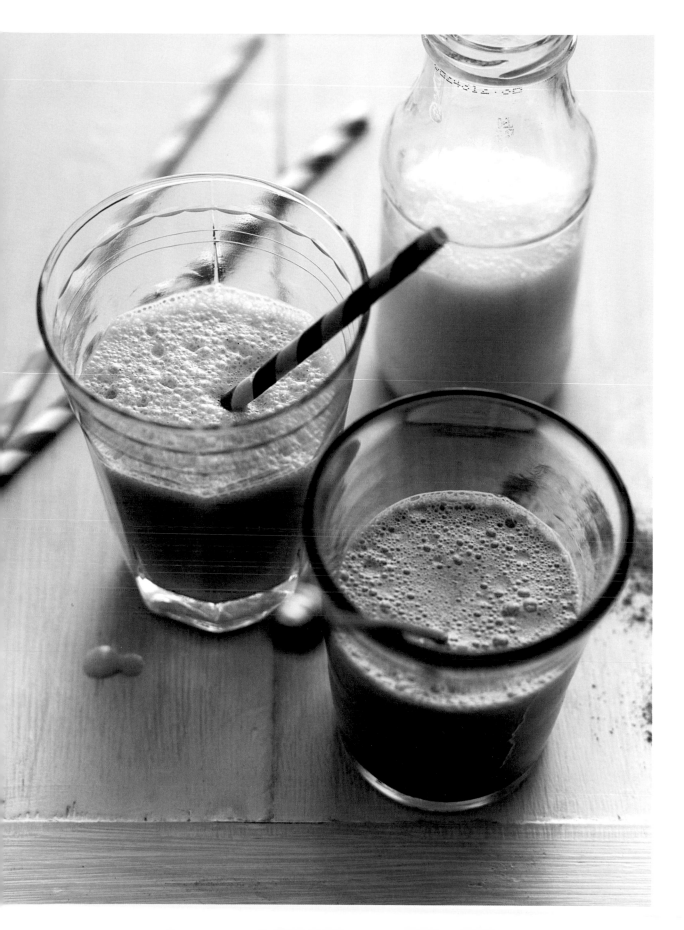

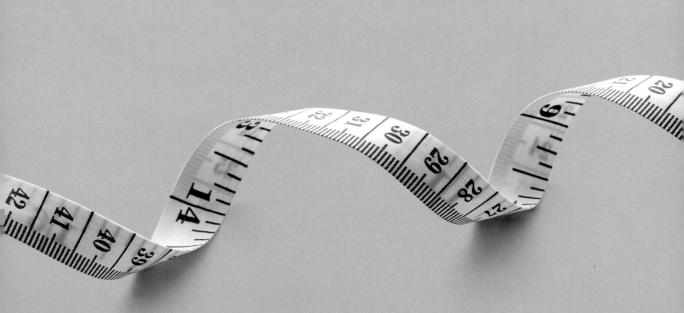

on the
high street

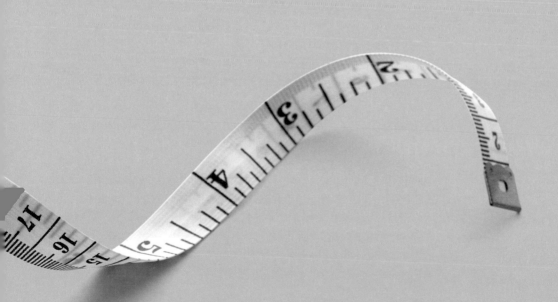

369
CALORIES
PER SERVING

chip shop fish

SERVES 4
PREP: 20 MINUTES
COOK: 20–25 MINUTES

1 litre sunflower oil,
   for deep-frying
2 tbsp plain flour
½ tsp fine sea salt
4 fish fillets, such as
   haddock, cod or hake
   (each about 200g)
lemon wedges, for
   squeezing

FOR THE BATTER
50g cornflour
100g plain flour
1 tsp paprika (not smoked)
½ tsp fine sea salt
175ml cold water

A national favourite, fish and chips are usually laden with calories and fat. For this recipe, I've developed a special batter that doesn't absorb so much of the oil but still remains crisp on the outside while the fish steams inside. Serve with oven-baked chips (see page 141) or a small portion of ready-prepared oven chips and fresh mushy peas (below).

To make the batter, mix the cornflour, plain flour, paprika and salt together in a large bowl. Make a well in the centre and stir in the water. Beat with a large metal whisk to make a smooth batter.

Fill a large, deep saucepan a third full with sunflower oil and heat to 190°C. It's important to use a cooking thermometer and check the temperature regularly. Do not allow the oil to overheat or leave hot oil unattended. (Alternatively, use an electric deep-fat fryer heated to 190°C.) Preheat the oven to 220°C/Fan 200°C/Gas 7.

Put the flour in a wide dish and season with the salt. Add the fish fillets, one at a time, and turn to coat them in the seasoned flour.

When the oil has reached the right temperature, stir the batter well. Take a floured fish fillet and dip it in the batter to thoroughly coat it. Lift it out with 2 forks and gently shake off the excess batter. Lower the fish gently into the hot oil. Watch out for splashes as the oil will be extremely hot. Cook for 1½ minutes then lift out with tongs and place on a rack over a large baking tray.

Pre-fry the other fish fillets in the same way. Bake all the fish together for 15 minutes or until golden, crisp and cooked through.

Fresh mushy peas: Melt 15g butter in a saucepan and gently fry 1 small chopped onion and 1 crushed garlic clove for 3–4 minutes, or until softened, stirring. Add 250g frozen peas and 100ml of chicken stock. Boil for 3–4 minutes or until the peas are tender. Blitz using a stick blender until as smooth as possible. Season and serve warm. Serves 4. Calories per serving: 75

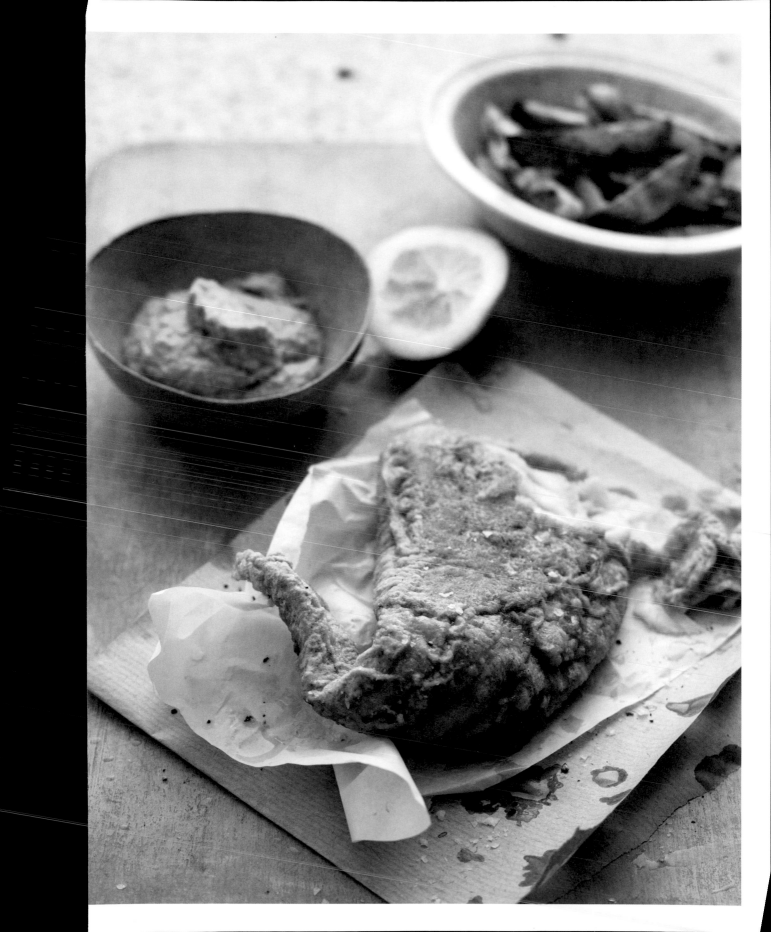

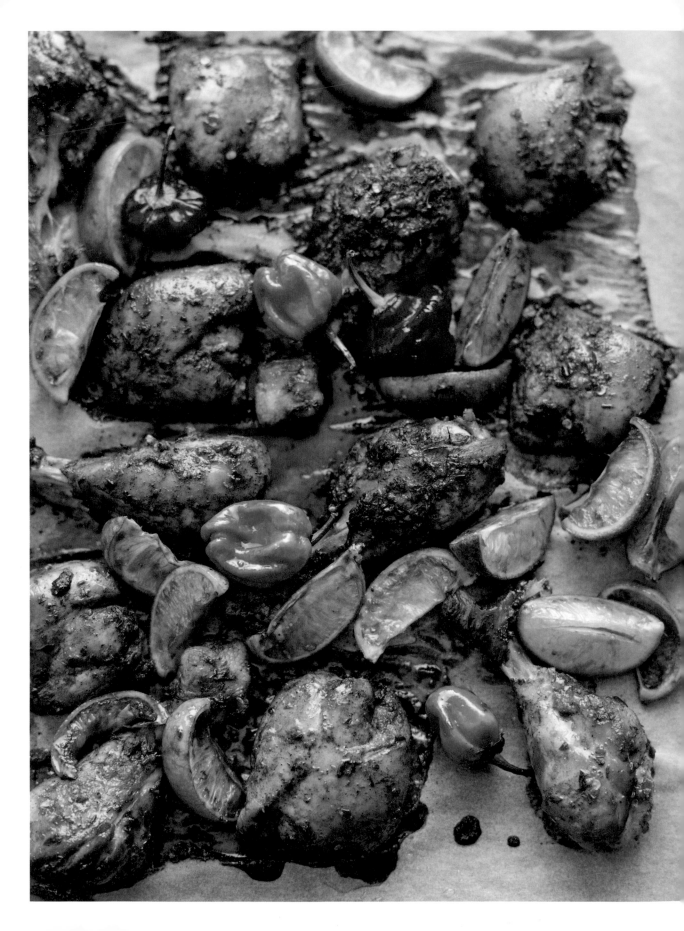

272
CALORIES
PER SERVING

jerk chicken

SERVES 4
PREP: 20 MINUTES
COOK: 25 MINUTES

6 chicken drumsticks
6 boneless, skinless chicken
 thighs (about 500g)
lime wedges and whole
 scotch bonnet chillies,
 to serve (optional)

FOR THE MARINADE
4 spring onions,
 roughly chopped
4 garlic cloves, halved
3 scotch bonnet or 2 red
 bird's eye chillies,
 stalks removed
25g chunk fresh root
 ginger, peeled and
 roughly chopped
4 tbsp dark soft
 brown sugar
3 tbsp fresh lime juice
2 tbsp dark soy sauce
1 tbsp fresh thyme leaves
1½ tsp ground allspice
1½ tsp ground mixed spice

Freeze the marinated
uncooked chicken in zip-
seal bags for up to 1 month.
Thaw overnight in the fridge
and cook as the recipe.

Tip: If you can't find scotch
bonnet chillies, use red
bird's eye chillies instead.

Sweet and spicy, this chicken is deliciously messy and moreish. It freezes beautifully and would be great served cold for a picnic, perhaps with coleslaw (see page 154) or a crisp green salad.

To make the marinade, put all the ingredients in a small food processor and blitz to a thick purée. You will need to remove the lid and push the mixture down a couple of times with a rubber spatula until the right consistency is reached. Put into a large bowl.

Put the chicken drumsticks on a board and ease the skin off. Trim off as much fat as possible from the drumsticks and thighs and slash each one a couple of times with a sharp knife and put them in the bowl with the marinade. Cover and leave to marinate in the fridge for at least 2 hours.

Preheat the oven to 220°C/Fan 200°C/Gas 7. Line a large baking tray with baking parchment and place the chicken on top.

Bake the chicken for 30–35 minutes or until thoroughly cooked and deep golden brown. Turn after 15 minutes and add the lime wedges and whole chillies to the tray, if using. Serve hot or cold with the lime wedges for squeezing. Don't eat the chillies whole as they are extremely spicy! Cut into thin slices and serve sprinkled on top if you like. (Remember to wash your hands after preparing the chillies.)

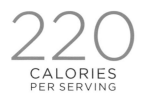

220

CALORIES
PER SERVING

piri piri chicken

Unlike the chicken from some restaurants, these chicken breasts are packed with spices without being covered in oil. This makes a really lovely fresh supper when served with a big salad and my lovely piri piri sauce – you'll find the recipe on page 168. Perfect for freezing too.

SERVES 4
PREP: 15 MINUTES
COOK: 20–25 MINUTES

4 boneless, skinless chicken breasts (each about 175g)
oil, for spraying or brushing
1 large red onion, cut into thin wedges
4 short cherry tomato vines

PIRI PIRI MARINADE
3 red bird's eye chillies, sliced
3 garlic cloves, halved
20g fresh flat-leaf parsley
4 tbsp fresh lemon juice
2 tbsp red wine vinegar
2 tsp sweet smoked paprika
1 tsp dried oregano
1 tsp caster sugar
1 tsp flaked sea salt

Freeze the marinated, uncooked chicken in zip-seal bags for up to 1 month. Defrost overnight in the fridge and cook as the recipe.

To make the marinade, put the chillies, garlic, parsley with its stalks, lemon juice, vinegar, paprika, oregano, sugar and salt in a small food processor and blitz until well combined and chopped up very finely.

Slash each chicken breast 3–4 times with a knife and place in a large, non-metallic bowl. Pour over the marinade and turn the chicken until well coated. Cover the dish with cling film, then leave to marinate in the fridge for at least 4 hours or ideally overnight.

Preheat the oven to 210°C/Fan 190°C/Gas 6½. Take the chicken out of the bowl and place it on a lightly oiled baking tray. Roast the chicken for 10 minutes before adding the red onion and tomatoes and cook for another 10 minutes or until lightly browned and cooked through (there should be no pinkness remaining).

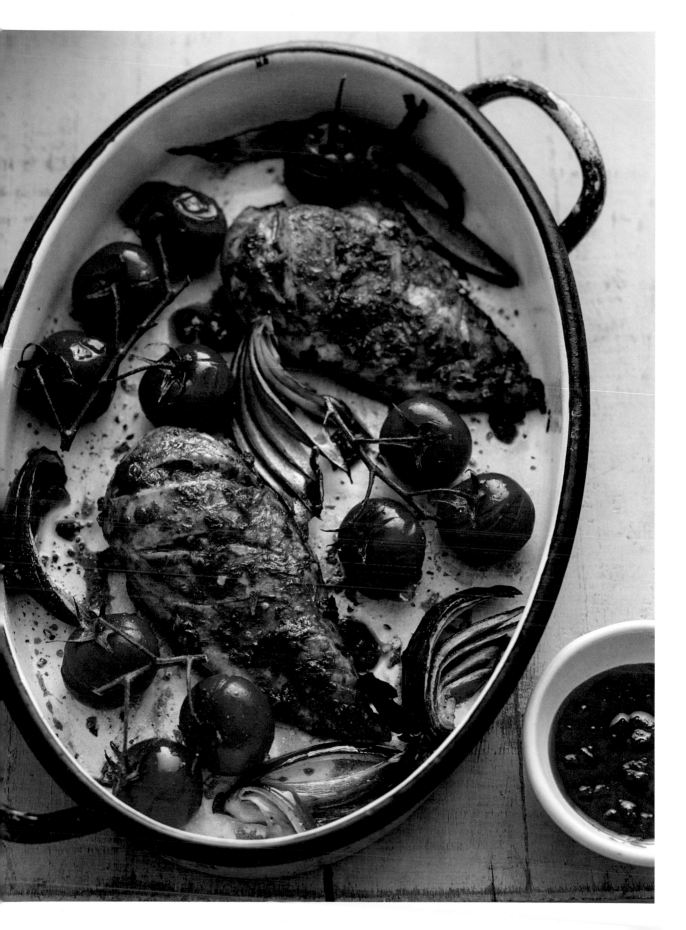

352

giant cornish pasty

SERVES 8
PREP: 30 MINUTES,
PLUS RESTING TIME
COOK: 45 MINUTES

FOR THE PASTRY
400g plain flour,
    plus extra for rolling
2 tsp baking powder
50g butter, chilled
    and cubed
50g lard, chilled
    and cubed
200ml lukewarm water
beaten egg, to glaze
ground black pepper

FOR THE FILLING
100g potato, peeled
    and cut into roughly
    1cm cubes
150g swede, peeled
    and cut into roughly
    1cm cubes
1 small onion, finely
    chopped
225g lean frying steak
1½ tbsp plain flour
flaked sea salt
ground black pepper

Freeze the pasty by
wrapping cooled slices
tightly in foil and putting
them into a zip-seal bag.
Freeze for up to 1 month.
Thaw overnight in the fridge
and serve cold or reheat
in the microwave.

This hearty pasty is great for a picnic or packed lunches, served warm or cold. By making one giant pasty rather than individual pastries, you don't need to use so much pastry and it's a lot quicker. Use kitchen scissors to snip the meat instead of chopping it – seems a bit odd at first but it works.

To make the filling, put the potato, swede and onion in a large mixing bowl and season with salt and plenty of black pepper.

Trim the steak of any hard fat or gristle, slice into 5mm strips, then snip very carefully with kitchen scissors until as finely chopped as possible. Put the steak in a second bowl. Season with more salt and lots more pepper. Toss with the flour until evenly coated.

For the pastry, put the flour and baking powder in a large bowl and rub in the butter and lard until the mixture looks like fine breadcrumbs. Stir in the water and mix to a smooth dough.

Turn the dough out onto a floured surface and knead lightly. Divide the pastry in half. Take one half and flatten slightly. Roll out to a circle roughly 28cm in diameter, turning the pastry a quarter-turn every couple of rolls to keep it round. Lift the pastry over the rolling pin and onto a baking tray lined with baking parchment. Roll the other piece of pastry into a circle roughly 30cm in diameter.

Mix the vegetables and meat together, then spoon the mixture onto the round of pastry on the baking tray, piling it up slightly towards the centre and leaving a 4cm empty border around the edge of the pastry. Brush around the empty border very lightly with a little beaten egg. Cover with the other circle of pastry, press the edges together firmly and trim neatly with a sharp knife. Crimp or press with a fork to seal. Brush with more egg to glaze and chill in the fridge for 30 minutes.

Preheat the oven to 180°C/Fan 160°C/Gas 4. Sprinkle the pasty lightly with black pepper, then bake for 45 minutes. Leave to stand at room temperature for 5 minutes before serving.

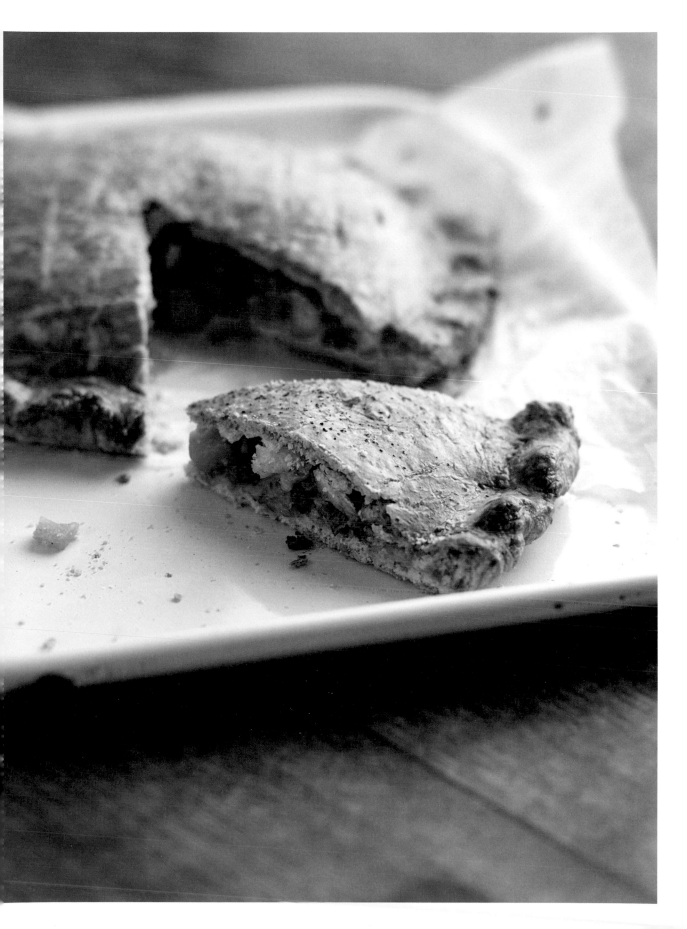

352
CALORIES
PER SERVING

portobello mushroom and halloumi 'burger'

SERVES 4
PREP: 20 MINUTES
COOK: 10 MINUTES

4 sourdough bread slices
½ garlic clove
250g pack halloumi
   cheese, cut into 8 slices
4 large Portobello
   mushrooms, stalks
   removed
1 little gem lettuce,
   leaves separated
1 large tomato, sliced

FOR THE PIRI PIRI SAUCE
2 tbsp fresh lemon juice
1 tbsp tomato purée
1 tbsp crushed chillies
   (from a jar)
2 garlic cloves, crushed
1 tsp sweet smoked paprika
1 tsp dried oregano
1 tbsp extra virgin olive oil
½ tsp flaked sea salt
ground black pepper

Freeze the sauce in small zip-seal bags for up to 1 month. Defrost at room temperature for about 1 hour. The cheese and mushrooms are best not frozen.

Tip: If you have a large griddle pan, you may have room for the mushrooms as well as the cheese. Place on top 2–3 minutes before the cheese and turn once or twice as they cook.

This veggie 'burger' will have even determined meat-eaters asking for the recipe, not least because of the fab piri piri sauce served alongside it. Halloumi is a unique, semi-firm Cypriot cheese that can be sliced and grilled without melting too much. Its salty taste and firm texture really complements the earthiness of the mushrooms.

Preheat the oven to 200°C/Fan 180°C/Gas 6. Place the mushrooms, stalk side down, on a baking tray and cook for 10 minutes or until tender.

Place a griddle pan over a high heat for about 5 minutes or until very hot. While the griddle pan is heating, make the sauce. Whisk the lemon juice with the tomato purée, chillies, garlic, smoked paprika, oregano, salt and lots of black pepper in a small bowl. Whisk in the oil and leave to stand.

Toast the bread slices on the hot griddle until lightly browned, then rub with the garlic and place on 4 plates. Put the sliced halloumi on the griddle and cook for 1–2 minutes on each side or until hot and lightly charred. Top the toast with lettuce and sliced tomato, then add the hot mushroom and cheese. Drizzle with the piri piri sauce and serve.

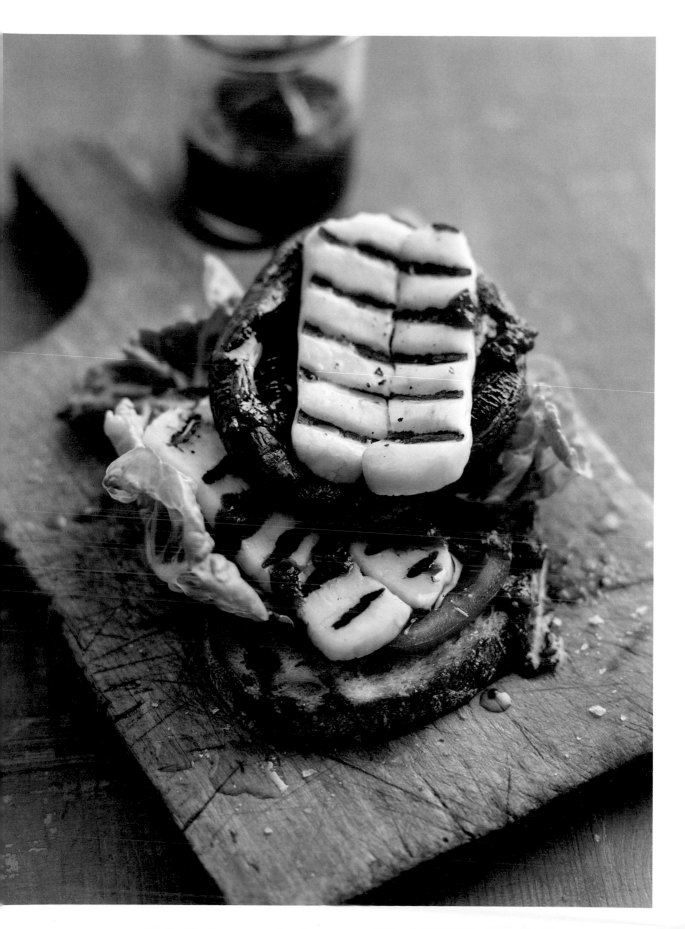

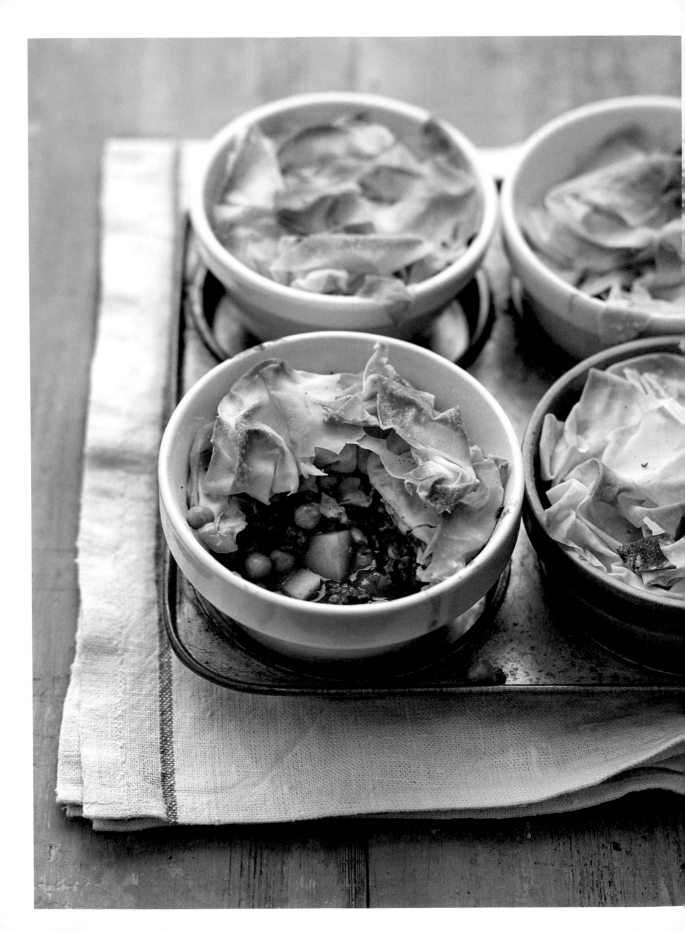

231
CALORIES
PER SERVING

minced beef
and onion pies

MAKES 6
PREP: 15 MINUTES
COOK: 50–55 MINUTES

300g potatoes, peeled and
   cut into roughly 1cm dice
2 medium onions,
   finely chopped
250g lean minced beef
1 tbsp tomato ketchup
1 tbsp brown sauce
1 tbsp Worcestershire sauce
1 tbsp plain flour
300ml beef stock, made
   with 1 beef stock cube
100g frozen peas
6 filo pastry sheets
   (each about 45g)
flaked sea salt
ground black pepper

Freeze the unbaked pies
until solid then cover with
foil and freeze for up to
3 months. Defrost in the
fridge overnight before
baking as the recipe.

Warm and filling, these pies make a wonderful winter dinner
for the family and contain fewer calories than the high street
versions. Try making extra and freezing them for when you
need a proper pie fix.

Bring a medium saucepan of water to the boil, add the
potatoes and return to the boil. Cook for 1 minute. Drain
and set aside.

Place a large non-stick saucepan over a high heat and fry
the onions and minced beef together for 2–3 minutes or until
the beef is no longer pink, stirring to break up the mince as
you cook. Reduce the heat and add the tomato ketchup, brown
sauce, Worcestershire sauce and flour. Cook for 1 minute, then
slowly stir in the stock. Season with a good pinch of salt and
lots of black pepper.

Cover the pan loosely with a lid, bring to a gentle simmer
and cook for 25–30 minutes, or until the beef is tender and
the sauce is thick, stirring occasionally. Add the par cooked
potatoes and the frozen peas. Leave to cool for 20 minutes.

Preheat the oven to 200°C/Fan 180°C/Gas 6. Divide the mince
between six individual pie dishes. Spray one of the filo pastry
sheets with a little oil and scrunch up loosely on top of a pie.
Repeat with the rest of the pastry and pies. Bake for 20 minutes
or until the filling is hot and the pastry is golden and crisp on top.

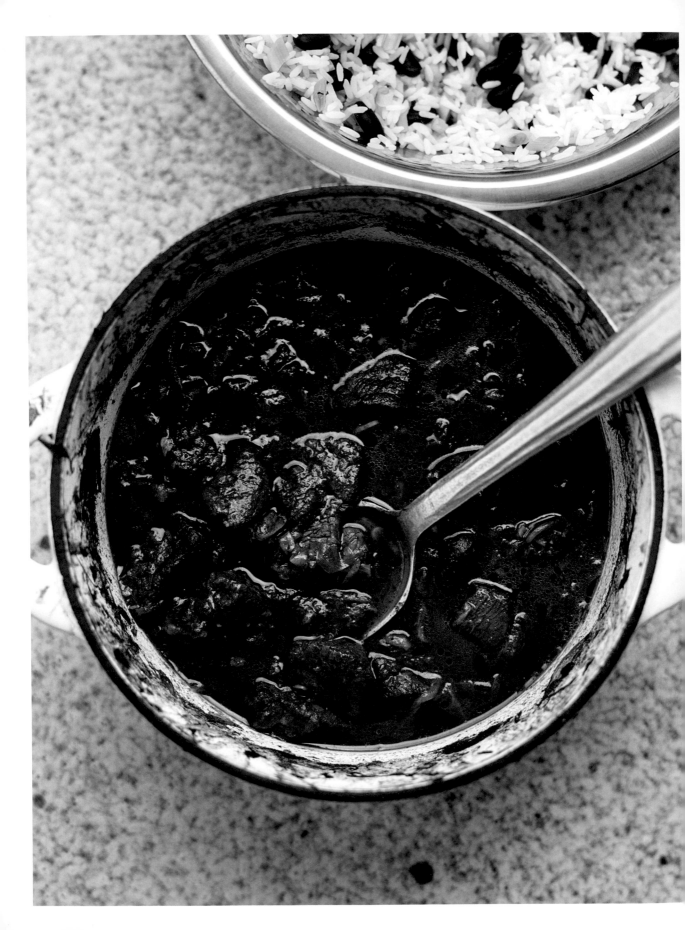

368
CALORIES
PER SERVING

caribbean lamb curry

SERVES 6

**PREP: 30 MINUTES,
PLUS MARINATING TIME**

COOK: 2–2½ HOURS

1.2kg lean lamb leg steaks
   (or boneless lamb
   leg meat)
3 tbsp red wine vinegar
1 tbsp fresh thyme leaves
2 tsp ground allspice
1 tsp ground cloves
2 tbsp medium curry
   powder
1 tsp flaked sea salt
1 tbsp sunflower oil
1 large onion, thinly sliced
4 garlic cloves, thinly sliced
1 scotch bonnet chilli, finely
   chopped (deseed first
   if you like)
400g can chopped
   tomatoes
2 tbsp tomato purée
2 tbsp dark soft brown
   sugar
ground black pepper

Freeze the curry in a large
freezer-proof container for
up to 2 months. Defrost in
the fridge overnight and
reheat thoroughly in a large
saucepan, stirring regularly
until piping hot.

Tip: Take care to wash
your hands really well after
handling the chilli or wear
latex gloves to prepare it.

**Really flavourful and hot but not too fiery, feel free to adjust
the chilli to suit your taste. This is a fairly saucy curry so a small
portion of rice tossed with canned red kidney beans or frozen
peas suits it well.**

Trim the lamb of any hard fat and sinew and cut into roughly
3–4cm chunks. Put the lamb in a medium bowl with the vinegar,
thyme, allspice, cloves, curry powder, salt and lots of black
pepper. Mix well and leave to marinate in the fridge for
30 minutes.

Preheat the oven to 180°C/Fan 160°C/Gas 4. Heat the oil in a
large non-stick flameproof casserole and gently fry the onion,
garlic and chilli for 5 minutes, while stirring. You may want to
turn on your extractor fan as the chilli could make you cough.
Stir in the lamb pieces and cook for 3 minutes or until lightly
coloured all over.

Add the canned tomatoes, tomato purée and sugar. Refill
the tomato can with cold water and stir the water into the
casserole. Bring to a simmer, cover with a lid and transfer
to the oven. Cook for 1½–2 hours or until very tender,
stirring halfway through the cooking time.

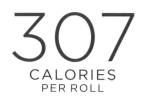

307 CALORIES PER ROLL

jumbo sausage rolls

MAKES 6
PREP: 30 MINUTES, PLUS COOLING TIME
COOK: 25–30 MINUTES

1 tsp sunflower oil
2 medium onions, finely chopped
1 garlic clove, crushed
300g lean minced pork
3 tbsp dried breadcrumbs
10g fresh sage, leaves finely chopped
½ tsp ground mace or nutmeg
320g reduced-fat ready-rolled puff pastry sheet
1 tbsp plain flour, for rolling
beaten egg, to glaze
flaked sea salt
ground black pepper

Open freeze the uncooked but glazed sausage rolls, then put them into a freezer-proof container, seal and freeze for up to 3 months. Defrost in the fridge and cook as the recipe, adding an extra 5 minutes or until cooked throughout.

Another lighter version of a classic that doesn't sacrifice the meaty taste of pork and sage in order to save calories. Let your family taste them before telling them the 'lower calorie' secret – I bet they won't notice.

Heat the oil in a small non-stick saucepan and gently fry the onions and garlic for 5 minutes or until well softened, stirring regularly. Scrape everything into a bowl and leave to cool.

Add the minced pork, breadcrumbs, sage and the mace or nutmeg to the bowl. Season with a good pinch of salt and plenty of black pepper and mix well. Preheat the oven to 200°C/Fan 180°C/Gas 6. Line a large baking tray with baking parchment.

Roll out the pastry on a lightly floured surface so the short ends are about 30cm wide, then cut it into 3 equal strips. Place one-third of the sausage meat down the centre of one of the pastry strips, leaving a gap around the edge. Lightly brush the edge with beaten egg.

Bring one egged side over the meat, then bring the other egged side up and over. Turn the roll over, cut it in half and place it, seam-side down, on the prepared baking tray. Repeat with the other pastry strips and remaining sausage meat.

Slash the top of each roll a few times, brush with beaten egg, then bake for about 20–25 minutes or until golden and cooked through.

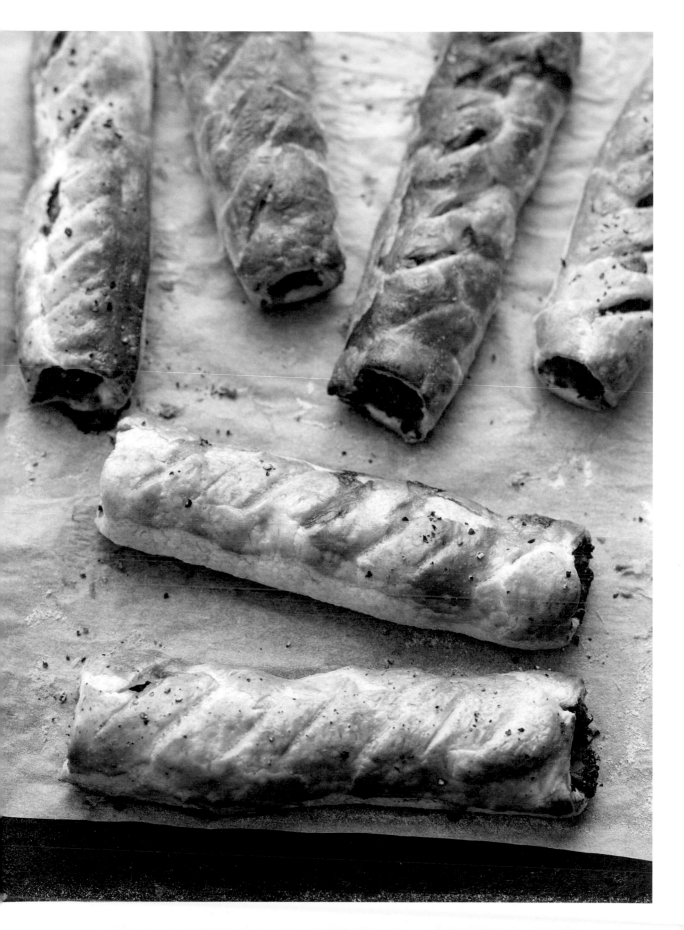

a few notes on the recipes

INGREDIENTS

Where possible, choose free-range chicken, meat and eggs. Eggs used in the recipes are medium unless otherwise stated.

All poultry and meat has been trimmed of as much hard or visible fat as possible, although there may be some marbling within the meat. Boneless, skinless chicken breasts weigh around 175g. Fish has been scaled, gutted and pin-boned, and large prawns are deveined. You'll be able to buy most fish and seafood ready prepared but ask your fishmonger if not and they will be happy to help.

PREPARATION

Do as much preparation as possible before you start to cook. Discard any damaged bits, and wipe or wash fresh produce before preparation unless it's going to be peeled.

Onions, garlic and shallots are peeled unless otherwise stated, and vegetables are trimmed. Lemons, limes and oranges should be well washed before the zest is grated. Weigh fresh herbs in a bunch, then trim off the stalks before chopping the leaves. I've used medium-sized vegetables unless stated. As a rule of thumb, a medium-sized onion and potato (such as Maris Piper) weighs around 150g.

All chopped and sliced meat, poultry, fish and vegetable sizes are approximate. Don't worry if your pieces are a bit larger or smaller than indicated, but try to keep to roughly the size so the cooking times are accurate. Even-sized pieces will cook at the same rate, which is especially important for meat and fish.

I love using fresh herbs in my recipes, but you can substitute frozen herbs in most cases. Dried herbs will give a different, more intense flavour, so use them sparingly.

The recipes have been tested using sunflower oil, but you can substitute vegetable, groundnut or mild olive oil. I use dark soy sauce in the test kitchen but it's fine to use light instead – it'll give a milder flavour.

CALORIE COUNTS

Nutritional information does not include the optional serving suggestions. When shopping, you may see calories described as kilocalories on food labels; they are the same thing.

HOW TO GET THE BEST RESULTS

Measuring with spoons

Spoon measurements are level unless otherwise stated. Use a set of measuring spoons for the best results; they're endlessly useful, especially if you're watching your sugar, salt or fat intake.

    1 tsp (1 teaspoon) = 5ml
    1 dsp (1 dessertspoon) = 10ml
    1 tbsp (1 tablespoon) = 15ml

A scant measure is just below level and a heaped measure is just above. An Australian tablespoon holds 20ml, so Australian cooks should use three level teaspoon measures instead. See page 179 for more measurement conversions.

HOW TO FREEZE

Freezing food will save you time and money, and lots of the dishes in this book freeze extremely well. If you don't need all the servings at the same time, freeze the rest for another day. Where there are no instructions for freezing a dish, freezing won't give the best results once reheated.

When freezing food, it's important to cool it rapidly after cooking. Separate what you want to freeze from what you're going to serve and place it in a shallow, freezer-proof container. The shallower the container, the quicker the food will cool (putting it in the freezer while it's still warm will raise the freezer temperature and could affect other foods). Cover loosely, then freeze as soon as it's cool.

If you're freezing a lot of food at once, for example after a bulk cooking session or a big shop, flip the fast freeze button on at least two hours before adding the new dishes and leave it on for twenty-four hours afterwards. This will reduce the temperature of your freezer and help ensure that food is frozen as rapidly as possible.

When freezing food, expel as much air as possible by wrapping it tightly in a freezer bag or foil to help prevent icy patches, freezer burn and discolouration, or flavour transfer between dishes. Liquids expand when frozen, so leave a 4–5cm gap at the top of containers.

If you have a small freezer and need to save space, flat-freeze thick soups, sauces and casseroles in strong zip-seal freezer bags. Fill the bag halfway, then turn it over and flatten it until it is around 1–2cm thick, pressing out as much air as possible and sealing firmly.

Place delicate foods such as breaded chicken or fish fillets and burgers on a tray lined with baking parchment, and freeze in a single layer until solid before placing in containers or freezer bags. This method is called open freezing and helps stop foods sticking together in a block, so you can grab what you need easily.

Label everything clearly, and add the date so you know when to eat it at its best. I aim to use food from the freezer within about four months.

DEFROSTING

For the best results, most foods should be defrosted slowly in the fridge for several hours or overnight. For safety's sake, do not thaw dishes at room temperature.

Flat-frozen foods (see above) will thaw and begin to reheat at almost the same time. Just rinse the bag under hot water and break the mixture into a wide-based pan. Add a dash of water and warm over a low heat until thawed. Increase the heat, adding a little more water if necessary, and simmer until piping hot throughout.

Ensure that any foods that have been frozen are thoroughly cooked or reheated before serving.

CONVERSION CHARTS
Oven temperature guide

	Electricity °C	Electricity °F	Electricity (fan) °C	Gas Mark
Very cool	110	225	90	$\frac{1}{4}$
	120	250	100	$\frac{1}{2}$
Cool	140	275	120	1
	150	300	130	2
Moderate	160	325	140	3
	170	350	160	4
Moderately hot	190	375	170	5
	200	400	180	6
Hot	220	425	200	7
	230	450	210	8
Very hot	240	475	220	9

Liquid measurements

Metric	Imperial	Australian	US
25ml	1fl oz		
60ml	2fl oz	$\frac{1}{4}$ cup	$\frac{1}{4}$ cup
75ml	3fl oz		
100ml	3$\frac{1}{2}$fl oz		
120ml	4fl oz	$\frac{1}{2}$ cup	$\frac{1}{2}$ cup
150ml	5fl oz		
180ml	6fl oz	$\frac{3}{4}$ cup	$\frac{3}{4}$ cup
200ml	7fl oz		
250ml	9fl oz	1 cup	1 cup
300ml	10$\frac{1}{2}$fl oz	1$\frac{1}{4}$ cups	1$\frac{1}{4}$ cups
350ml	12$\frac{1}{2}$fl oz	1$\frac{1}{2}$ cups	1$\frac{1}{2}$ cups
400ml	14fl oz	1$\frac{3}{4}$ cups	1$\frac{3}{4}$ cups
450ml	16fl oz	2 cups	2 cups
600ml	1 pint	2$\frac{1}{2}$ cups	2$\frac{1}{2}$ cups
750ml	1$\frac{1}{4}$ pints	3 cups	3 cups
900ml	1$\frac{1}{2}$ pints	3$\frac{1}{2}$ cups	3$\frac{1}{2}$ cups
1 litre	1$\frac{3}{4}$ pints	1 quart or 4 cups	1 quart or 4 cups
1.2 litres	2 pints		
1.4 litres	2$\frac{1}{2}$ pints		
1.5 litres	2$\frac{3}{4}$ pints		
1.7 litres	3 pints		
2 litres	3$\frac{1}{2}$ pints		

essential extras

Here's my list of suggested 50–150 calorie foods that you can use to supplement the 123 Plan. All calories per serving listed here are approximate; a few wayward calories here and there won't make a difference to your allowance. See page 6 for more information on essential extras and how they fit into the plan. I've also listed some 'free' vegetable ideas, of which you can eat as much as you like! Make sure your plate is half filled with vegetables or salad, or serve them in a large bowl on the side. Eating more greens will help fill you up and provide lots of extra nutrients in your diet. Your skin will look better and the weight should drop off.

50 CALORIES PER SERVING

30g (about 5) ready-to-eat dried apricots
15g (1 tbsp) light mayo
30g (2 tbsp) hummus
40g drained artichoke antipasti in oil
60g whole olives

4 fresh apricots
200g fresh blackberries
200g fresh blackcurrants
100g fresh cherries
2 clementines or satsumas
100g fresh figs
½ grapefruit
85g grapes
2 kiwis
100g fresh mango
200g melon
1 medium nectarine
1 medium orange
1 medium peach
1 medium pear
125g fresh pineapple
100g canned pineapple in juice
2 plums
200g papaya
100g pomegranate seeds
200g raspberries
200g strawberries

100g fresh tomato salsa
50g tzatziki
1 level tbsp orange marmalade
1 level tbsp mango chutney
1 level tsp taramasalata
1 level tbsp honey

2cm slice (about 20g) ciabatta
1 x 10g rye crispbread, such as Ryvita
50g cooked puy lentils, green lentils
1 x measure (25ml) spirits (light or dark, e.g. rum, vodka)

1 tbsp single cream
1 tbsp half-fat crème fraiche
10g Parmesan
30g soft French goat's cheese
25g (1½ tbsp) light soft cheese
150ml orange juice (not from concentrate)
100ml regular soy milk
100g low-fat natural yoghurt
50g (about 3 wafer thin slices) of ham, turkey or chicken

75 CALORIES PER SERVING

150ml semi-skimmed milk
100g low-fat cottage cheese
25g (small wedge) Camembert
1 tbsp double cream
1 tbsp crème fraiche
50g ricotta cheese
¼ 125g ball of fresh mozzarella

¼ average avocado (35g)
50g smoked salmon
1 rasher back bacon, grilled or dry-fried
50g cooked, skinless chicken breast
100g cooked jumbo prawns (about 9)

1 medium apple
100g blueberries
25g dried mango

2 cream crackers
20g rice cakes (2 or 3)
20g plain breadsticks (about 4)
½ English muffin
1 slice medium white or brown bread
15g shop-bought (not takeaway) prawn crackers
1 oatcake

½ 160g tin tuna in brine, drained
40g sun-dried (or sun-blush) tomatoes in oil, drained
30g (2 tbsp) raisins
1 medium egg, boiled

100 CALORIES PER SERVING

1 large egg
40g feta cheese
100g plain cottage cheese
50g (2½ tbsp) soured cream
25g blue cheese
100ml fresh custard
25g cooking chorizo
30g ready-to-eat chorizo
   (about 5 thin slices)
25g salami (about 5 thin
   slices)
1 heaped tbsp pesto

45g Parma ham
   (about 3 slices)
30g smoked mackerel fillet
1 medium banana

1 level tbsp peanut butter
1 tbsp extra virgin olive oil
30g popping corn kernels
20g unsalted plain cashews
20g tortilla chips
25g wasabi peas

20g plain crisps

1 slice of thick cut bread
½ plain bagel
1 x 45g soft white bread roll
½ regular pitta bread
1 slice German style rye bread
1 crumpet
120g baked beans
45g dried couscous
30g dried wholewheat pasta
25g dried soba noodles
30g dried quinoa

125ml wine (white, red, rose)
125ml sparkling wine/
   Champagne
½ pint lager
½ pint bitter
½ pint dry cider

150 CALORIES PER SERVING

35g Cheddar cheese
100g skinless chicken breast,
   baked or grilled

100g cooked brown rice
115g cooked easy-cook white
   rice
40g dried basmati rice
1 potato, baked, boiled or
   mashed without fat
   (195g raw weight)
130g baked sweet potato
   (about ½ large potato)
40g dried rice noodles
50g dried egg noodles
100g cooked pasta
40g porridge oats
50g shop-bought naan bread
   (about ½)

25g unsalted almonds
175ml wine (not sparkling)

'FREE' SAUCES

Brown sauce, in moderation;
   each tbsp is 24 calories
Fish sauce (nam pla)
Ketchup, in moderation;
   each tbsp is 20 calories
Horseradish sauce
Hot sauce (Tabasco)
Mint sauce (not jelly)
Mustard, any variety
   (English, Dijon,
   wholegrain, American)
Soy sauce
Vinegars (balsamic,
   white wine, malt, etc.)
Worcestershire sauce

Any herbs or spices

'FREE' VEGETABLES

Artichokes, including tinned
   hearts (but not in oil)
Asparagus
Aubergine
Baby sweetcorn
Beans, any green (not baked)
   (French, runner, etc.)
Bean sprouts
Beetroot, fresh, cooked
   or pickled
Broccoli
Brussels sprouts
Butternut squash
Cabbage, all kinds
   (savoy, red, white)
Carrots
Cauliflower
Celeriac
Celery
Chicory
Chillies, including pickled
   jalapeños
Cornichons
Courgettes
Cucumber
Fennel
Garlic
Kale
Leeks
Lemons
Limes
Lettuce and salad greens
   (watercress, baby
   spinach, romaine)
Mangetout
Marrow
Mushrooms
Onions
Peppers
Pickled onions
Radishes
Shallots
Spring onions
Sugar snap peas
Swede
Tomatoes, including tinned
   (but not sun-dried)
Turnips

nutritional information
per serving

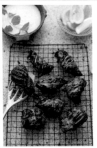

page 10 / serves 4
tandoori chicken

210 energy (kcal)
891 energy (kJ)
44.3 protein (g)
3.9 carbohydrate(g)
2.0 fat (g)
0.6 saturated fat (g)
0.1 fibre (g)
3.2 sugars (g)

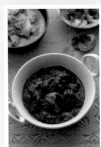

page 12 / serves 4
my favourite chicken tikka masala

291 energy (kcal)
1225 energy (kJ)
45.7 protein (g)
13.0 carbohydrate (g)
6.6 fat (g)
1.0 saturated fat (g)
4.2 fibre (g)
8.5 sugars (g)

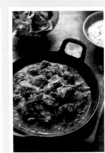

page 14 / serves 6
creamy chicken passanda

297 energy (kcal)
1244 energy (kJ)
38.2 protein (g)
8.2 carbohydrate (g)
12.6 fat (g)
4.2 saturated fat (g)
1.0 fibre (g)
6.5 sugars (g)

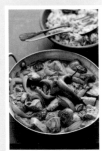

page 16 / serves 4
chicken jalfrezi

279 energy (kcal)
1179 energy (kJ)
44.6 protein (g)
13.2 carbohydrate (g)
5.7 fat (g)
1.1 saturated fat (g)
4.0 fibre (g)
11.9 sugars (g)

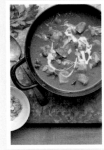

page 18 / serves 4
chicken korma

323 energy (kcal)
1356 energy (kJ)
45.0 protein (g)
15.2 carbohydrate (g)
9.2 fat (g)
2.6 saturated fat (g)
2.3 fibre (g)
11.3 sugars (g)

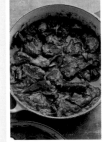

page 20 / serves 6
lamb rogan josh

375 energy (kcal)
1569 energy (kJ)
43.6 protein (g)
9.3 carbohydrate (g)
18.4 fat (g)
7.2 saturated fat (g)
3.2 fibre (g)
7.5 sugars (g)

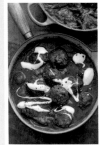

page 22 / serves 4
lamb meatball curry

335 energy (kcal)
1398 energy (kJ)
26.2 protein (g)
19.5 carbohydrate (g)
17.2 fat (g)
7.2 saturated fat (g)
2.2 fibre (g)
7.0 sugars (g)

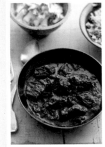

page 24 / serves 6
simple beef madras

342/18* energy (kcal)
1435/75* energy (kJ)
45.6/1.7* protein (g)
7.8/2.7* carb (g)
14.4/0.1* fat (g)
5.1/0* saturated fat (g)
1.7/0.3* fibre (g)
6.4/2.4* sugars (g)
*cucumber raita

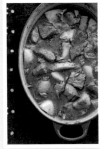

page 26 / serves 6
pork vindaloo with potatoes

364 energy (kcal)
1534 energy (kJ)
47.9 protein (g)
23.5 carbohydrate (g)
9.0 fat (g)
2.6 saturated fat (g)
2.9 fibre (g)
3.8 sugars (g)

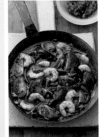

page 28 / serves 2
king prawn balti

214 energy (kcal)
899 energy (kJ)
21.3 protein (g)
16.3 carbohydrate (g)
7.3 fat (g)
0.9 saturated fat (g)
4.4 fibre (g)
13.7 sugars (g)

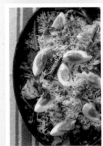

page 30 / serves 6
vegetable biryani

284 energy (kcal)
1186 energy (kJ)
12.6 protein (g)
41.3 carbohydrate (g)
7.8 fat (g)
1.6 saturated fat (g)
6.3 fibre (g)
9.7 sugars (g)

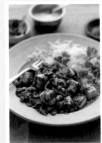

page 32 / serves 4
mutter paneer

312 energy (kcal)
1299 energy (kJ)
18.6 protein (g)
16.3 carbohydrate (g)
19.3 fat (g)
10.9 saturated fat (g)
5.0 fibre (g)
10.8 sugars (g)

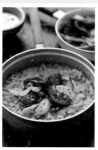

page 34 / serves 4
mixed vegetable dhal

236 energy (kcal)
1002 energy (kJ)
13.6 protein (g)
40.7 carbohydrate (g)
3.3 fat (g)
0.5 saturated fat (g)
7.7 fibre (g)
10.3 sugars (g)

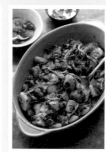

page 36 / serves 4
channa masala

216 (kcal)
911 energy (kJ)
11.0 protein (g)
30.3 carbohydrate (g)
6.6 fat (g)
0.7 saturated fat (g)
9.0 fibre (g)
8.9 sugars (g)

page 38 / serves 4
light saag aloo

189 energy (kcal)
797 energy (kJ)
6.0 protein (g)
34.8 carbohydrate (g)
3.8 fat (g)
0.4 saturated fat (g)
6.2 fibre (g)
7.5 sugars (g)

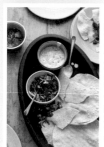

page 40 / serves 1
poppadums with tomato and onion salad

74/27* energy (kcal)
311/114* energy (kJ)
4.5/2.1* protein (g)
13.8/4.7* carb (g)
1.1/0.1* fat (g)
0.2/0* saturated fat (g)
2.6/0* fibre (g)
1.9/4.5* sugars (g)
*minted yoghurt sauce

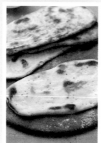

page 42 / serves 8
skinny naan bread

155 energy (kcal)
659 energy (kJ)
5.3 protein (g)
31.4 carbohydrate (g)
1.8 fat (g)
0.5 saturated fat (g)
1.6 fibre (g)
2.8 sugars (g)

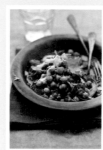

page 46 / serves 4
sesame prawn toasts

118 energy (kcal)
494 energy (kJ)
6.2 protein (g)
4.2 carbohydrate (g)
8.8 fat (g)
1.2 saturated fat (g)
0.8 fibre (g)
0.4 sugars (g)

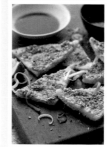

page 48 / serves 4
vegetable spring rolls

187/30* energy (kcal)
781/129 energy (kJ)
4.7/0* protein (g)
29.8/7.5* carb (g)
4.3/0* fat (g)
0.5/0* saturated fat (g)
2/0* fibre (g)
4.5/7.5* sugars (g)
*chilli and garlic sauce

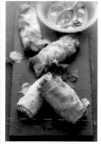

page 50 / serves 4
shredded duck wraps with hoisin sauce

115/217* energy (kcal)
483/899* energy (kJ)
10.9/9.7* protein (g)
8.2 carbohydrate (g)
4.4/16.3* fat (g)
1.3/4.8* saturated fat (g)
1.3 fibre (g)
2.5 sugars (g)
*with skin

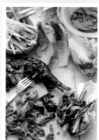

page 52 / serves 4
dim sum

244 energy (kcal)
1040 energy (kJ)
14 protein (g)
38 carbohydrate (g)
5.2 fat (g)
1.6 saturated fat (g)
2.0 fibre (g)
0.8 sugars (g)

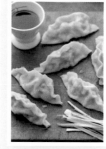

page 54 / serves 4
special chow mein

327 energy (kcal)
1381 energy (kJ)
36.4 protein (g)
36.8 carbohydrate (g)
3.7 fat (g)
0.8 saturated fat (g)
5.4 fibre (g)
13.7 sugars (g)

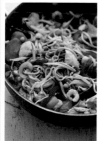

page 56 / serves 4
chicken and sweetcorn soup

134 energy (kcal)
561 energy (kJ)
13.0 protein (g)
13.0 carbohydrate (g)
3.6 fat (g)
0.9 saturated fat (g)
1.2 fibre (g)
1.2 sugars (g)

page 58 / serves 4
kung po chicken with broccoli

289 energy (kcal)
1218 energy (kJ)
37.2 protein (g)
14.0 carbohydrate (g)
8.4 fat (g)
1.5 saturated fat (g)
3.1 fibre (g)
9.7 sugars (g)

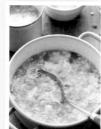

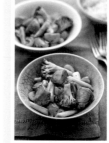

page 60 / serves 4
beef with green peppers in black bean sauce

225 energy (kcal)
943 energy (kJ)
26.9 protein (g)
10.6 carbohydrate (g)
7.7 fat (g)
2.4 saturated fat (g)
3.2 fibre (g)
7.5 sugars (g)

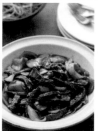

page 62 / serves 4
chilli beef stir-fry

217 energy (kcal)
911 energy (kJ)
24.2 protein (g)
9.2 carbohydrate (g)
8.4 fat (g)
2.3 saturated fat (g)
2.0 fibre (g)
6.9 sugars (g)

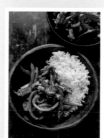

page 64 / serves 4
sweet and sour pork

284 energy (kcal)
1201 energy (kJ)
29.5 protein (g)
30.1 carbohydrate (g)
5.8 fat (g)
1.9 saturated fat (g)
3.5 fibre (g)
27.0 sugars (g)

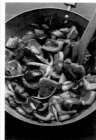

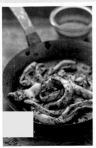

page 66 / serves 4
salt and pepper squid

77 energy (kcal)
324 energy (kJ)
11.6 protein (g)
1.5 carbohydrate (g)
2.8 fat (g)
0.5 saturated fat (g)
0 fibre (g)
0 sugars (g)

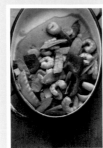

page 68 / serves 2
king prawn stir-fry with vegetables

272 energy (kcal)
1144 energy (kJ)
23.2 protein (g)
29.8 carbohydrate (g)
7.2 fat (g)
1.0 saturated fat (g)
8.8 fibre (g)
14.8 sugars (g)

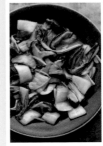

page 70 / serves 4
stir-fried pak choi with mushrooms

58 energy (kcal)
241 energy (kJ)
2.5 protein (g)
7.1 carbohydrate (g)
2.1 fat (g)
0.2 saturated fat (g)
1.7 fibre (g)
1.3 sugars (g)

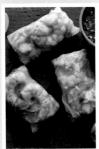

page 74 / serves 4
vietnamese summer rolls

225 energy (kcal)
945 energy (kJ)
18.3 protein (g)
34.5 carbohydrate (g)
1.5 fat (g)
0.3 saturated fat (g)
2.7 fibre (g)
8.1 sugars (g)

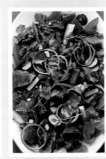

page 76 / serves 4
fragrant beef, herb and watermelon salad

265 energy (kcal)
1113 energy (kJ)
24.6 protein (g)
23.8 carbohydrate (g)
8.3 fat (g)
2.7 saturated fat (g)
3.8 fibre (g)
21.2 sugars (g)

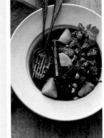

page 78 / serves 4
beef massaman curry

495 energy (kcal)
2077 energy (kJ)
48.1 protein (g)
30.8 carbohydrate (g)
20.7 fat (g)
10.6 saturated fat (g)
3.6 fibre (g)
6.6 sugars (g)

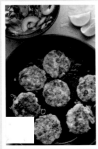

page 80 / serves 4
thai fishcakes

146 energy (kcal)
612 energy (kJ)
21.1 protein (g)
7.3 carbohydrate (g)
3.7 fat (g)
0.5 saturated fat (g)
0.4 fibre (g)
0.8 sugars (g)

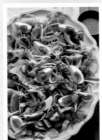

page 82 / serves 6
gado-gado chicken salad

238/67* energy (kcal)
999/279* energy (kJ)
27.6/2.0* protein (g)
16.8/2.8* carb (g)
7.1/5.3* fat (g)
1.9/2.0* saturated fat (g)
4.0/0* fibre (g)
6.4/0.8* sugars (g)
*peanut dressing

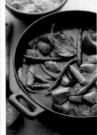

page 84 / serves 4
thai red chicken curry

306 energy (kcal)
1287 energy (kJ)
45.1 protein (g)
12.0 carbohydrate (g)
8.7 fat (g)
6.2 saturated fat (g)
4.2 fibre (g)
8.1 sugars (g)

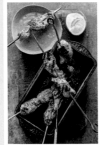

page 86 / serves 4
simple chicken satay

174/53* energy (kcal)
31.8/221* energy (kJ)
0.9/1.7* protein (g)
0.9/2.9* carbohydrate (g)
4.8/3.9* fat (g)
0.9/1.0* saturated fat (g)
0.0/0.0* fibre (g)
0.6/0.5* sugars (g)
*satay sauce

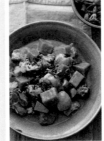

page 88 / serves 4
penang chicken and sweet potato curry

355/48* energy (kcal)
1495/203* energy (kJ)
36.9/3.2* protein (g)
22.3/3.9* carb (g)
13.7/2.4* fat (g)
7.5/0.3* saturated fat (g)
3.3/3.6* fibre (g)
7.3/3.0* sugars (g)
*stir-fried broccoli

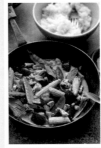

page 90 / serves 2
jungle curry

331 energy (kcal)
1393 energy (kJ)
48.3 protein (g)
12.1 carbohydrate (g)
10.1 fat (g)
1.5 saturated fat (g)
6.1 fibre (g)
9.0 sugars (g)

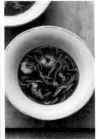

page 92/ serves 4
prawn noodle broth

179 energy (kcal)
750 energy (kJ)
14.4 protein (g)
27.3 carbohydrate (g)
1.0 fat (g)
0.1 saturated fat (g)
1.3 fibre (g)
4.0 sugars (g)

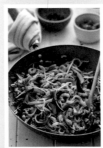

page 94 / serves 4
pad thai with prawns

331 energy (kcal)
1383 energy (kJ)
19.4 protein (g)
39.4 carbohydrate (g)
10.4 fat (g)
2.0 saturated fat (g)
1.7 fibre (g)
6.3 sugars (g)

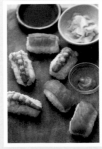

page 98 / serves 4
hand-pressed nigiri sushi

144 energy (kcal)
606 energy (kJ)
9 protein (g)
25.5 carbohydrate (g)
0.6 fat (g)
0.3 saturated fat (g)
4.2 fibre (g)
3.9 sugars (g)

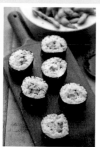

page 100 / serves 4
maki sushi rolls

218/134* energy (kcal)
918/561* energy (kJ)
7.6/11.5* protein (g)
37.2/8.9* carb (g)
4.2/6.1* fat (g)
0.9/0.8* saturated fat (g)
7.9/0* fibre (g)
1.9/4.3* sugars (g)
*edamame (serves 2)

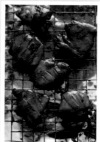

page 102 / serves 4
teriyaki chicken

259 energy (kcal)
1090 energy (kJ)
37.1 protein (g)
12.3 carbohydrate (g)
4.9 fat (g)
1.4 saturated fat (g)
0.0 fibre (g)
12.2 sugars (g)

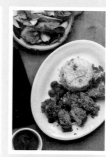

page 104 / serves 4
chicken katsu curry

300 energy (kcal)
1267 energy (kJ)
47.1 protein (g)
19.1 carbohydrate (g)
4.4 fat (g)
1.1 saturated fat (g)
1.6 fibre (g)
7.6 sugars (g)

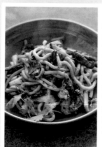

page 106 / serves 2
ginger chicken with udon noodles

475 energy (kcal)
2000 energy (kJ)
48.8 protein (g)
41.0 carbohydrate (g)
12.3 fat (g)
2.5 saturated fat (g)
0.5 fibre (g)
2.9 sugars (g)

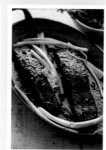

page 108/ serves 4
sticky miso salmon

308 energy (kcal)
1284 energy (kJ)
31.6 protein (g)
5.3 carbohydrate (g)
17.4 fat (g)
2.9 saturated fat (g)
0.2 fibre (g)
3.5 sugars (g)

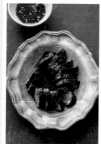

page 110 / serves 4
pork and ponzu dressing

203 energy (kcal)
853 energy (kJ)
28.4 protein (g)
3.1 carbohydrate (g)
5.5 fat (g)
1.8 saturated fat (g)
0.1 fibre (g)
2.7 sugars (g)

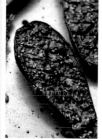

page 112 / serves 2
miso ginger aubergines

172 energy (kcal)
722 energy (kJ)
6.9 protein (g)
20.2 carbohydrate (g)
4.0 fat (g)
0.5 saturated fat (g)
6.8 fibre (g)
13.0 sugars (g)

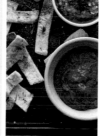

page 116 / serves 6
red pepper hummus and pitta crisps

133 energy (kcal)
565 energy (kJ)
5.7 protein (g)
23.7 carbohydrate (g)
2.4 fat (g)
0.3 saturated fat (g)
3.4 fibre (g)
2.6 sugars (g)

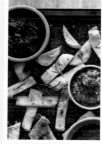

page 117 / serves 6
baba ganoush

30/46* energy (kcal)
131/194* energy (kJ)
1.3/2.0* protein (g)
2.1/5.6*carb (g)
2.1/1.9* fat (g)
0.3/0.3* sat fat (g)
2.6/1.3* fibre (g)
1.8/5.2* sugars (g)
*minted beetroot dip

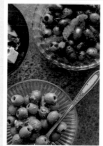

page 118 / serves 4
moroccan marinated olives

63/71* energy (kcal)
260/290* energy (kJ)
0.5/0.9* protein (g)
1.2/0.2* carb(g)
6.2/7.3* fat (g)
0.9/1.2* sat fat (g)
1.5/1.4* fibre (g)
0.7/0* sugars (g)
*pesto olives

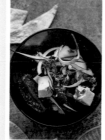

page 118 / serves 4
feta and tomatoes

92/43* energy (kcal)
384/181* energy (kJ)
4.0/1.0* protein (g)
3.8/9.0* carb (g)
6.8/0.5* fat (g)
2.6/0.1* saturated fat (g)
0.2/0.5* fibre (g)
0.8/0.2* sugars (g)
*tortilla chips

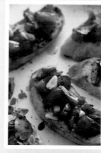

page 120 / serves 2
tomato and basil bruschetta

162/163* energy (kcal)
683 /683*energy (kJ)
4.4/4.7* protein (g)
21.2/16.3* carb(g)
7.2/9.3* fat (g)
1.1/4.3* saturated fat (g)
3.3/2.4* fibre (g)
6.2/1.2* sugars (g)
*mushroom topping

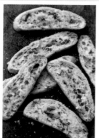

page 122 / serves 6
garlic and herb bread

141 energy (kcal)
591 energy (kJ)
3.6 protein (g)
17.4 carbohydrate (g)
6.9 fat (g)
3.6 saturated fat (g)
1.2 fibre (g)
1.2 sugars (g)

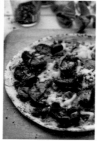

page 124 / serves 2
pizza pronto

337 energy (kcal)
1410 energy (kJ)
16.9 protein (g)
44.2 carbohydrate (g)
10.5 fat (g)
3.9 saturated fat (g)
5.7 fibre (g)
1.3 sugars (g)

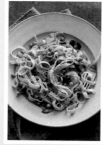

page 126 / serves 4
creamy pasta carbonara

440 energy (kcal)
1845 energy (kJ)
26.3 protein (g)
41.1 carbohydrate (g)
18.9 fat (g)
9.0 saturated fat (g)
3.6 fibre (g)
2.0 sugars (g)

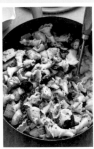

page 128 / serves 4
**pollo pasta
with pesto**

498 energy (kcal)
2094 energy (kJ)
31.6 protein (g)
48.1 carbohydrate (g)
19.9 fat (g)
5.4 saturated fat (g)
0.6 fibre (g)
1.0 sugars (g)

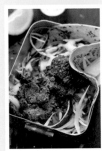
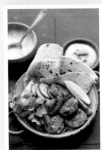

page 130 / serves 4
lamb doner kebabs

298 energy (kcal)
1252 energy (kJ)
22.3 protein (g)
26.8 carbohydrate (g)
12.0 fat (g)
4.9 saturated fat (g)
1.7 fibre (g)
2.6 sugars (g)

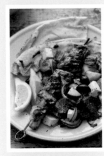

page 132 / serves 4
chicken shish kebab

419 energy (kcal)
1767 energy (kJ)
39.8 protein (g)
43.1 carbohydrate (g)
10.7 fat (g)
3.1 saturated fat (g)
5.1 fibre (g)
7.1 sugars (g)

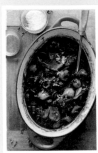

page 134 / serves 6
stifado

344 energy (kcal)
1442 energy (kJ)
45.4 protein (g)
4.5 carbohydrate (g)
13.5 fat (g)
5.1 saturated fat (g)
1.9 fibre (g)
4.2 sugars (g)

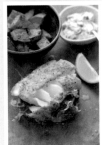

page 136 / serves 4
falafel

260 energy (kcal)
1098 energy (kJ)
10.3 protein (g)
43.6 carbohydrate (g)
5.8 fat (g)
0.9 saturated fat (g)
6 fibre (g)
2.1 sugars (g)

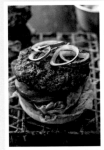

page 140 / serves 4
lower fat burgers

321/119* energy (kcal)
1347/505* energy (kJ)
31.4/3* protein (g)
20.5/25* carb (g)
13.2/1* fat (g)
5.5/0.1* sat fat (g)
2.8/2.6* fibre (g)
6.0/0.9* sugars (g)
*oven-baked chips

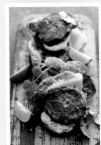

page 142 / serves 4
spicy bean burgers

190/45* energy (kcal)
803/187* energy (kJ)
10.4/0.5* protein (g)
31.7/1.1* carb (g)
3.2/4.4* fat (g)
0.4/1.7* sat fat (g)
9.6/0* fibre (g)
5.2/0.9* sugars (g)
*lime and coriander
mayo

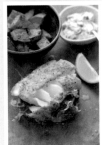

page 144 / serves 4
**fish burgers with
tartare sauce**

270/34* energy (kcal)
1141/143* energy (kJ)
32.3/1.1* protein (g)
28.5/2.3* carb (g)
3.7/2.4* fat (g)
0.7/0.4* saturated fat (g)
1.3/0.7* fibre (g)
1.1/1.5* sugars (g)
*tartare sauce

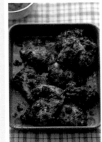

page 146 / serves 4
**southern-style
chicken**

352 energy (kcal)
1486 energy (kJ)
55.2 protein (g)
15.0 carbohydrate (g)
8.3 fat (g)
2.5 saturated fat (g)
0.7 fibre (g)
2.6 sugars (g)

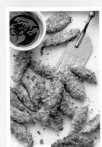

page 148 / serves 4
crispy chicken strips

337 energy (kcal)
1427 energy (kJ)
47.6 protein (g)
27.4 carbohydrate (g)
4.9 fat (g)
1.1 saturated fat (g)
0.4 fibre (g)
1.4 sugars (g)

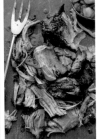

page 150 / serves 6
smoky pulled pork

354/66* energy (kcal)
1480/279* energy (kJ)
39.0/0.3* protein (g)
4.2/17.2* carb (g)
20.4/0.1* fat (g)
6.7/0 saturated fat (g)
0/1.9* fibre (g)
4.2/17.2 sugars (g)
*apple sauce

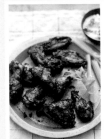

page 152 / serves 4
**buffalo wings with
blue cheese dip**

390 energy (kcal)
1630 energy (kJ)
31.2 protein (g)
13.0 carbohydrate (g)
24.1 fat (g)
9.1 saturated fat (g)
0.2 fibre (g)
12.8 sugars (g)

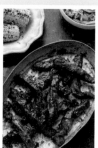

page 154 / serves 4
**sticky pork 'ribs'
in barbecue sauce**

225/81* energy (kcal)
950/339* energy (kJ)
33.9/3.6* protein (g)
10.6/6.9* carb (g)
5.5/4.5* fat (g)
1.8/0.7* saturated fat (g)
0.2/2.8* fibre (g)
10.4/6.1* sugars (g)
*coleslaw

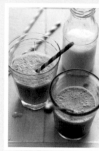

page 156 / serves 1
strawberry milkshake

136/160*/141** energy (kcal)
572/674/598* energy (kJ)
6.5/6.6*/4.6** protein (g)
16.1/21.1*/27.9** carb(g)
5.4/5.9*/2.0** fat (g)
3.4/3.8*/1.2** sat fat (g)
0.7/0*/1.5** fibre (g)
15.6/20.4*/25.6** sugars (g)
*chocolate milkshake
**banana milkshake

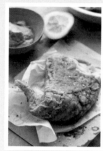

page 160 /serves 4
chip shop fish

369/75* energy (kcal)
1554/314* energy (kJ)
39.4/3.8* protein (g)
30.3/7.1* carb (g)
10.1/3.7* fat (g)
1.3/2.1* sat fat (g)
1.2/4.6* fibre (g)
0.4/2.5*sugars (g)
*fresh mushy peas

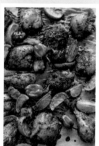

page 162 / serves 4
jerk chicken

272 energy (kcal)
1147 energy (kJ)
37.9 protein (g)
12.2 carbohydrate (g)
8.5 fat (g)
2.3 saturated fat (g)
0.3 fibre (g)
11.5 sugars (g)

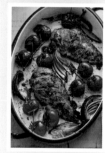

page 164 / serves 4
piri piri chicken

220 energy (kcal)
932 energy (kJ)
43.3 protein (g)
6.6 carbohydrate (g)
2.3 fat (g)
0.6 saturated fat (g)
1.9 fibre (g)
5.5 sugars (g)

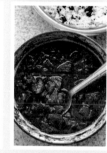

page 166 / serves 8
giant cornish pasty

352 energy (kcal)
1478 energy (kJ)
12.8 protein (g)
46.3 carbohydrate (g)
14.1 fat (g)
6.6 saturated fat (g)
3.1 fibre (g)
2.3 sugars (g)

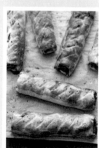

page 168 / serves 4
**portobello mushroom
and halloumi 'burger'**

352 energy (kcal)
1474 energy (kJ)
19.2 protein (g)
25.3 carbohydrate (g)
19.4 fat (g)
11.2 saturated fat (g)
2.9 fibre (g)
3.8 sugars (g)

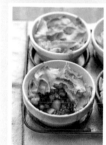

page 170 / serves 6
**minced beef
and onion pies**

231 energy (kcal)
975 energy (kJ)
14.2 protein (g)
32.7 carbohydrate (g)
5.2 fat (g)
1.9 saturated fat (g)
3.1 fibre (g)
5.2 sugars (g)

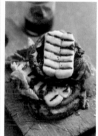

page 172 / serves 6
caribbean lamb curry

368 energy (kcal)
1539 energy (kJ)
42.0 protein (g)
9.8 carbohydrate (g)
18.0 fat (g)
7.2 saturated fat (g)
1.6 fibre (g)
8.3 sugars (g)

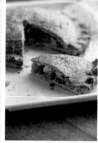

page 174 / serves 6
jumbo sausage rolls

307 energy (kcal)
1286 energy (kJ)
14.4 protein (g)
30.9 carbohydrate (g)
14.5 fat (g)
6.3 saturated fat (g)
1.0 fibre (g)
3.1 sugars (g)

index

First published in Great Britain in 2015
by Orion Publishing Group Ltd
Carmelite House, 50 Victoria Embankment,
London EC4Y 0DZ
An Hachette UK Company

10 9 8 7 6 5 4 3

Text © Justine Pattison 2015
Design and layout © Orion 2015

A CIP catalogue record for this book is available
from the British Library.
ISBN: 978 1 4091 5473 0

Designer: Smith & Gilmour
Photographer: Cristian Barnett
Props stylist: Claire Bignell
Creative director: Justine Pattison
Nutritional analysis calculated by: Lauren Brignell
Recipe assistants: Kirsty Thomas, Vanessa Graham
Kitchen assistants: Jess Blain, Emily PB
Project editor: Jillian Young
Copy editor: Elise See Tai
Proofreader: Mary-Jane Wilkins
Indexer: Rosemary Dear

Printed and bound in Italy

*Every effort has been made to ensure that the
information in this book is accurate. The information
will be relevant to the majority of people but may not
be applicable in each individual case, so it is advised
that professional medical advice is obtained for
specific health matters. Neither the publisher nor
author accept any legal responsibility for any personal
injury or other damage or loss arising from the use or
misuse of the information in this book. Anyone making
a change in their diet should consult their GP,
especially if pregnant, infirm, elderly or under 16.*

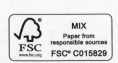

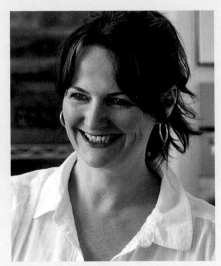

Acknowledgements

Firstly, huge thanks to everyone who enjoys my
recipes and the way I cook. You have given me such
fantastic feedback; I hope you like these dishes just
as much.

I'm truly grateful to the very talented photographer
Cristian Barnett for wonderful photographs that really
make my food come to life. And the brilliant Claire
Bignell for her superb creative skills, selecting the
perfect props and helping make the recipes look
both beautiful and achievable.

Massive thanks to Lauren Brignell for all her invaluable
nutritional support and the hundreds of recipes she has
analysed over the past few months. Also, thanks to the
extremely hard-working Kirsty Thomas and Vanessa
Graham for carefully testing the recipes and assisting
on shoot days. Your skill and input has been invaluable.

At Orion, I would like to thank Amanda Harris for
believing in this project right from the beginning and
for trusting me to get on and develop the series. Also
thank you to Jillian Young, my fantastic editor, for her
guidance and professionalism and Helen Ewing for
her design support.

A big thank you to everyone at Smith & Gilmour for
making the books look eye-catching, practical and
readable. I'm also grateful to my agent, Zoe King, at
The Blair Partnership, for her constant encouragement
and enthusiasm.

And, a final thank you to my family and friends:
Angela, Ann, Angie, Bella, Charlotte, Clare, Emma,
Michelle, Rachel, Sarah and Tamsin for their
unwavering support.

Thank you to Kitchen Aid for kindly lending me
their brilliant mixers, blenders and food processors
for recipe testing.